I0117728

USE MIND AND NOT FORCE: A TAIJI MEMOIR

Other works by the same author

Fiction
Ride a White Mare
Jade is My Stone
Splitting Apart
The Shades of Paracelsus
The Drain Brains

Nonfiction
TAO: Total Person and One World
Tales of the Dragon, the Bear and Other Wondrous Creatures

Verse
Mostly Friday Nights
Pick Up the Pearl

USE MIND AND NOT FORCE: A TAIJI MEMOIR

Patrick McGowan

Fomelhaut 2019

© Copyright Patrick McGowan
Typeset and printed by Patrick McGowan
m/s prepared on LibreOffice open source software
Fomelhaut Publishing, 2019
ISBN 978-0-9925812-5-1

twitter @_pjmcgowan
email: pat@pjmcgowan.com
copies available on amazon/kindle direct publishing
blog at www.pjmcgowan.com

To the next generation of explorers

'I must, before I die, find some way to say the essential thing that is in me, that I have never said yet - a thing that is not love or hate or pity or scorn, but the very breath of life, fierce and coming from far away, bringing into human life the vastness and the fearful passionless force of non-human things. — Bertrand Russell

Acknowledgments

In quoting and referencing outside sources within the text I implicitly acknowledge the many people who have been part of this discovery exercise. I thank them all. Let this book be my expression of thanks. As online resources operate these days, texts and extracts I mention here are easily sourced.

I thank Simon Lim and my many taiji colleagues and associates over the decades for their warm and generous friendship.

I thank Dr Merlinda Bobis, supervisor of my Master of Creative Arts major work, and who led the project, *The Transnational Story Hub: Between Self and Other,* which brought me back to the theory of phenomenology and its ongoing value as a research tool.

I thank Julie Bates and Natalie Chabin for reading final drafts of the book and sharing comments.

I also thank the Keira Writers Group (part of the South Coast Writers Centre) for their constructive comments on the readings of some chapters at our monthly manuscript meetings.

Thanks to Rubing, my wife, for her encouragement along the way, and also her ideas about the book cover.

Thanks to Анна Куликова (monstreh) via pixabay.com for the base cover image.

TABLE OF CONTENTS

Introduction

In taiji, we move softly to develop strength, a strength of both mind and body. I have a clear measure of how well I am doing taiji each day: the softer it is, the more like water it is, the better it is. To use softness to develop strength seems counter-intuitive for some, even laughable. But here is an art that has been tried and tested over eight hundred years, is ranked as the martial art *par excellence* in China and is today universally accepted as one of the crown jewels of Chinese culture. However, martial arts skill is only a by-product of taiji training. Taiji is an art of health and wellbeing. This art has served me, as a non-Chinese person, in many ways for decades now and is still going strong.

Lately I have felt the desire to share my experience of the art, and with this desire has been a wish to express it in a fresh and engaging way. So here is an account of a Western taiji enthusiast wanting to throw some light on this often inscrutable Chinese cultural phenomenon.

I have a Chinese friend whose father back in China was a hobbyist art collector. In the early 1950s in Beijing, this man had the opportunity to buy a few works of art, some old and others by well-known local artists who had established a name for themselves in the early years of the twentieth century. He labelled his paintings, left them in a box in his office behind his desk and thought very little about them for many years. One day, in the late seventies, he and members of his family were sorting through boxes in his office, they re-discovered the paintings and liked what they saw. So they took them home and hung a few of them on the walls of their apartment to add colour and decoration to an otherwise drab inner city Beijing accommodation.

We often become familiar with those things we see everyday and so it was with these paintings in that family home. They didn't think much about them, not even when the apartment suffered rain damage and some of the paintings became waterstained. It was in the early nineties when stories began to emerge about how the works of certain local artists were rapidly appreciating in value.

One work was a watercolour painting of bamboo by Zheng Bangqiao (1693-1765). There was always the lingering thought that, though it was great art, it may not be from the hand of Zheng Bangqiao. Forgery is a serious concern in the art world. Eventually, the family decided to have the painting verified and it was indeed proved to be authentic, and worth a lot more than when first acquired.

When my friend told me the above story about the art works hanging on their living room wall for many years with little consideration of their market value, I immediately thought of my taiji art. While I have taught taiji at various times over the decades in local outlets such as adult education colleges and so on, for me my taiji has mostly been a very personal journey. I do the taiji form in my backyard every morning and then focus on my daily activities. I have always done this from my days at university up until today, and even when I worked for the Australian government overseas.

That thought of the unrecognised value of the art hanging in my friend's apartment lingered on the walls of my mind for years. Could my taiji be seen similarly? Have I been taking this precious art for granted? Could it be of more social value than I realise? As I mark the milestone of having done taiji daily for forty years, I realise I have accumulated a lot more experience and understanding than I knew. And so I have decided I should tell my story of taiji. Thus there is a strong autobiographical component to this book, related to my unfolding taiji adventure.

My taiji teacher, Simon Lim, whom I met at the University of Sydney when I enrolled there in 1980, always encouraged me to write about taiji. I tried many times to put pen to paper, but it seemed so elusive. At home sitting at my desk with a blank piece of paper, I would stare and stare and struggle to get going. I did manage to complete a few general articles here and there. But I decided I was not yet ready to write about taiji in the way I really wanted. There was the question of the writing skill but also I wonder now if I was too much wanting to tell others what was good for them. Simon's advantage in presenting taiji was that people came to him, to either his classes, his clinic or his home, and so he had an audience who was ready to hear. But people are rarely receptive when someone wants to talk at them, or write at them, being a little too fanatic for anyone's liking. And that's how I felt my writing was for me at that time. There was also the question of wanting to tell my teacher's story, rather than my own.

Today, as I write these words, I am in a different place. I am sharing what I know, and this is my voice. As far as readers go, it's up to each reader whether it resonates with them or not. I'm happy to bring this story to the table with the hope that some readers may find it helpful in their own quest for happiness and their search for a place of being where their life can unfold more freely.

Taiji, in those early days of wanting to write, was very much an energy experience, one hard to grasp and capture in words. This is a truth of taiji: we can only go along with it, we can't hold onto it. In more recent times, I have written a few dozen articles and some poems about taiji with a sense of sharing the experience in my own words. The deepest taiji truth is that we only need to save one person in this life and if we save that one person we save the whole world.

I have learned over many years that all people have the spark within themselves that can lead them to health and happiness without the need for any teacher or guide. But of course it is wonderful to witness people finding health, happiness and solutions to all the challenges that life poses. This is what motivates most teachers, healers and helpers: to see people find themselves in a new and better place.

I have read many books on taiji over the years. They are fine as sources of information and I always enjoy discovering more about taiji. Many of the writings of the great taiji teachers over the centuries are terse, and even cryptic. There are not written for the general public. Many are written for long term students who understand the teacher's often idiosyncratic language and use of particular words and phrases. A lot of later commentaries are repetitive, maybe even dogmatic, as if there is a right way and a wrong way to do taiji. And many commentators spend time on their particular lineage which can be interesting in its fine detail but it goes against the general idea of taiji as always looking forwards. On top of all that is the issue of translation from one language into another, and indeed from one culture to another.

So I have finally embraced my teacher's advice and begun to write about my own taiji experience. And my contribution is a refreshing perspective on an otherwise very inward-looking art. This is the book. I want to say it all, hold nothing back. I don't intend to follow up with a sequel to tell the rest of the story. These days, people are too busy to be led along like that. This is my contribution to the world stock of good quality reading.

In 2010 I was part of a transnational creative writing project involving writers from the University of Vigo, Spain and the University of Wollongong, Australia. The project was called *The Transnational Story Hub: Between Self and Other*. It was a series of sharing stories and poems with writing colleagues across the world and responding, in turn, to the stories and poems of those distant colleagues. After these steps, we proceeded to draw conclusions and theorise about what we had been doing. This was a type of grassroots joint creative and theoretical exercise.

In seeking the best way to understand and theorise about what we had been doing in this cultural exchange, I turned to the philosophy of phenomenology. I had studied this subject at university some thirty years earlier so it was a re-discovery. Phenomenology is a philosophy which emerged in the early twentieth century as a way to see our world in a fresh and unfettered way. Western thinking has a lot of deeply embedded assumptions about our relationship with our world. I will explore these issues elsewhere in the book. But phenomenology begins with the assumption that we are beings in the world, and are forever part of the world we are exploring.

In summary, the phenomenologist begins all philosophical and scientific inquiry with the concept of Dasein or being in the world. It is relevant to mention this here, because in this work, I am not attempting to present a scientific account of taiji or a philosophical thesis. This is an exploration of taiji as a phenomenon, firstly in my own life, and also as a social and cultural phenomenon.

Phenomenology as a practice has some established ways of proceeding in its inquiries. The two important steps are: a) we seek to be open to the experience or phenomenon before we reflect upon it. Almost as if we watch and listen to the phenomenon for the first time. We allow it to speak to us. The next step is: b) once we have opened ourselves, we close in on the meaning of the phenomenon as it appears in our experience.

I have chosen the phenomenological approach in this study of taiji. For example, when we are later considering the story of the founder of taiji, we are not applying pre-determined either/or judgements of whether it is true or not true, but we are seeking to listen to what the story of the founder has to tell us. This approach is actually helpful in how we do our own taiji exercise. Phenomenology has even been described as a psychic technique of non-resistance: we engage with open ears, open eyes and an open mind with the phenomenon we are exploring. As it turns out, this fits in very well with the theme of our book, to use mind and not force. If you are interested, I have attached a fuller account of phenomenology as a research method at Appendix One.

In writing this book, I have also set myself the goal of creating sentences that do more than simply convey information. I want to write sentences that reinforce my key themes. These are sentences that convey the essence and even form of taiji in their construction. This is a new dimension to writing that both the reader and writer may enjoy.

For many years, in studying creative writing, I followed the novelist, theorist and philosopher William Gass (1924-2017), who held some unconventional perspectives on sentence theory. In short, he proposed that each sentence has a soul which gives it its own rhythm, its own perception, its own emotion, its own imagination and of course its own architecture. Gass was adept in the skilfully crafted sentence, some which became very long and winding. But they were always there to serve the narrative of his work, reinforcing the intentions and themes of his work as a whole. I am inspired by his effort to add new dimensions to the sentence and so, as I sculpt sentences that can reflect the various aspects of taiji, I confess to an experimental style of writing. So please be on the lookout for some of those bonza sentences for want of a better word.

1 The idea

'Use mind and not force' (in Chinese 用意不用力 yòng yì bù yòng lì) is a phrase drawn from a treatise on taiji called *The Ten Important Points* by Master Yang Chengfu (1883-1939). While the phrase refers specifically to the practice of taiji martial art, it is also helpful advice in a much broader sense: to reach our goals, we can benefit greatly by making better use of mind and depending less on force. Some who like the idea may go on and try some taiji exercise. It is a wonderful embodiment of the idea and I am sure they will enjoy it. But taiji physical exercise is not essential. It may be a good way to communicate the idea but the taiji idea can be expressed in many ways.

I enjoy both the taiji idea and taiji exercise, and I have done so for most of my life. I attended my first taiji class one week after my twenty-first birthday. However, in the process of writing this book I discovered that my life had been preparing me for taiji a long time before I ever arrived at that first class. It's easy to say this with hindsight. It's not so easy to know what we are experiencing at the time we are going through it. However, I do believe that we have a nonphysical guidance in our life even though we may not be aware of it, not always tuned to it. A lot of the time, we may have a feel for the new experiences and events that are on their way to us, but we are not generally good at interpreting those feelings. Being able to connect with this nonphysical guidance in our daily life and to better interpret what's happening to us in the now are some of the benefits of a better familiarity with the taiji idea.

I love doing taiji exercise alone each morning, performing taiji and meditating on it. I have also shared the taiji form to many people over many years, but I believe it is time for me to use the form of words to share my experience with other who could benefit from it but may not get around to doing the exercise itself.

Over those years, I have met numerous people of such different cultural backgrounds, different life experiences and different belief systems. After all, I do live in a multicultural country. Through the enormous diversity of people I have encountered over this time, I can see that, whoever I am with, we always have something in common. That's why we are together in the first place. This common ground is the spontaneous and natural result of any group of people which comes together with a shared intention, even as each group member has their own path to travel.

People will always view the world from their own perspective. As I have travelled to many places, communicated widely with many people, and studied and researched over the years, I have been enriched by the vastly different takes on life I have observed in others. In summary, each of us is blessed with a vision of both the grandeur of life and much delicious detail. The most complete life is where these two factors blend together harmoniously. However, I do still wonder whether a lot of us, being too quick to make judgements about the world with its apparent lacks and excesses, and too often feel burdened to set the world right, get that balance between the big and the small perspectives right.

I intend to use moments from my own life to illustrate various points that I wish to make about taiji. The first experience I will relate comes from my earliest years of school, around Second Grade, when I was seven years old. It was a Catholic school and we were in a stage of preparation for the sacrament of Holy Communion usually received in Second Grade. Being taught to pray was an important part of the curriculum. While at home, we were taught to say our morning prayers, our prayers before sleep, prayers before and after meals etc. And we were impressed with the central importance of faith. I guess I was an impressionable young child and so I faithfully said all my prayers as instructed.

I recall some nights before sleep saying my prayers and I figured that if I said my prayers hard enough, I could make Our Lady, the mother of Jesus Christ, appear before me. We learned in class that she had appeared to many people around the world over the years. So as I prayed, I would tense my hands, and tense my arms and shoulders, my whole body, even squeeze the muscles around my closed eyes as I said my Hail Mary's and my Our Father's. But no matter how hard I prayed, she didn't appear. On reflection now, I see that maybe I was operating with at least a few false assumptions. Somewhere along the line, I interpreted my school teachers as saying that prayer is about doing something. But I was not only trying to use action, I was assuming that the more action the better, and hence the force. How superstitious was that! Thankfully, I grew out of this phase.

But we do need to consider how we 'do' things, how we 'make' things happen. I have noticed on many occasions, some of us, in going after what we want, become our own worst enemies. We can either push so hard we cruel our own efforts, or we can hold ourselves back with unhelpful attitudes and false assumptions. This is why I treasure the opportunity to share what I have discovered about taiji. It could be so helpful to so many of us seeking to navigate our own lives.

A recurring issue I want to address is the common belief that so many of us see action alone as the key to solving many of the problems we see in the world. I do see action as a necessary ingredient to any answer to solving problems and achieving our goals, but it needs to be thoughtful and directed action, inspired action. We have seen with problems large and small, that when small problems become larger, we think the answer is more action and often more force. We fail to see our relationship to the problem and how we may actually be feeding the problem. Whether it is personal relationships or international terrorism, people often escalate conflict by mindless action. Taiji has always been about settling ourselves and having a clear view of the situation so that we can take that step of more inspired action.

To help explain with an example, I have vivid memories of the time I spent with my taiji teacher learning the principles of natural health at his weekend clinic conducted at his home in the eighties. He used natural physiotherapy as part of his treatment. Amongst many other ailments, he attracted so many people with back problems. And sadly, many of his patients often came to him as a last resort, after all other mainstream options, including surgery, had failed and the chronic pain remained. Over and over again, he would say to his patients: 'whether the other people you go to use light or strong massage, fancy equipment or techniques, or even scalpels and saws, they depend on using force against the body, but most of the time the problem is the energy flow, and once we get the energy in your body flowing, the physical components of the body will come back into alignment by themselves.' He would then do acupressure massage on various points along the back, points which were often congested, and just need a helping hand to relax and refresh as the energy in the body has its own impetus to flow. A helping hand, yes, though there is a rich theory about the healing hand as well. I will give a fuller account of my teacher's clinic in a later chapter.

And while my teacher could use this important moment in a person's life, a visit to his clinic, to communicate his natural attitude, to get them to use less force on the physical components of life, and to seek better relaxation and alignment so things in general could flow better, I am using a different framework, that of philosophy and metaphysics, to carry on his work of communicating the very simple message for us to easier on ourselves. For me, the essence of taiji is to use the mind to determine our direction and then seek more harmonious ways to move towards our results. It means dealing with obstacles in a different way.

The thought of us as a physical being trapped in a physical world is a very dark one, one ironically which could only be created by a person with a rich imagination. We all need to see beyond the physical. In this book, I describe this as having a 'metaphysic'. We all need a metaphysic, a way to see beyond the physical, of some description. I use the word metaphysic in a very general sense. Metaphysics as taught in academic circles might not be very useful. While it may be rich and engaging for some, it may not have much to offer us in our day to day living. Of course, people are forever coming up with their own unique metaphysic to guide them through life. I am happy to say that the taiji tradition is part of the greater tradition of dao philosophy that has such a sublime metaphysic, one that could be communicated and used in a very practical sense in the course of daily living.

Teacher and healer, Beverly Milne, in her book *Tai-chi Spirit and Essence*, says that those who have a deep understanding of taiji rarely write about it. She comments how few who are able to write have the perception and ability to communicate what she calls taiji's 'inner reality' in our culture. She does admit that bookshops do hold endless manuals and videos on how to do taiji, and some information about the history of the art, mostly incorrect, but they are all so repetitive they offer little to the eager student. She does however say that taiji is fertile ground for writing because of the new perspectives it can bring and the much needed inspiration for the next generation of explorers. It is with these comments in mind, that I approach this account of my personal taiji experience and the way it has influenced so many aspects of my life which may not be readily apparent to the outside observer.

2 Before

The stories of most lives conform to the three Aristotelian stages of beginning, middle and end. Before we enter the two latter stages, how often we wish it was childhood, childhood and more childhood. However we are all on a path of inevitable unfolding where many decisions seem to have been made before long we were even born.

Where efforts are made to impede the path of a child's growth, the result can actually become childhood, more childhood and only childhood in a very sad way. But the human spirit is indomitable and once the physical and mental restraints are unbuckled, unstrapped and cast aside, the development continues, a natural process spurred by a self-generating momentum that remains a mystery to most.

I was a shy child, self-conscious, and easily made afraid. That's how it was much of the time. I knew about fun and laughter, usually when alone or with others my own age, far away from the influence of adults. I'm still uncertain what was going through the minds of most adults around me as I was growing up, though I have pleasant enough memories of extended family and friends who treated others with an instinctive kindness. I have warm memories of my Mancunian grandmother who was a good one for odd sayings such as: 'There are many saints walking the streets of Sydney these days and most people would never know it.'

From my earliest days of television watching I had a fascination with offbeat subjects. I gave it my full attention to any program about the supernatural, paranormal, psychic matters, occult, magic, mind power, telepathy, ESP and so on. I was easily engrossed. I was also a big fan of those shows that demonstrated the powers of hypnosis. A person under hypnosis seemed to acquire new skills and strength after a few words being spoken. So the power of the mind has always been a matter of interest to me. I have intuitively been formulating the principle of 'use mind and not force' from a very early age. But when I pointed out to others how marvelous these subjects were, I was met with vague interest or something more dismissive, with none of the fire that was alight in me.

My father, Gerald, sun sign in Libra, a man of cheerful disposition though sometimes prone to worry, a person who values social harmony and one with a strong sense of justice and balance that works as a neat bullshit detector, worked for many years as a salesman, firstly of insurance and then of real estate. He later ran several small businesses such as a newsagency and a cafe in partnership with my mother, Mary. Mary was a full-time housewife with her Virgoan flair for being tidy, organised and efficient in raising six children, before she applied those same innate skills to the family businesses.

I lived my formative years in the Sydney suburb of Campbelltown under a Catholic umbrella. My friends, my parents' friends, and the friends of my brothers and sisters mostly shared this background. Much of it was Irish Catholic with its talk of original sin, Jesus being so generous that he gave up his life to save ours, the power of the priest to bestow us with God's blessings and His holy sacraments and to forgive us of our inevitable sins.

My great-grandfather, John McGowan, arrived in Melbourne from Ireland in 1888 and he went on to raise a family, one of whose offspring was my grand-father, Jack McGowan, born in Beechworth in 1900. So I was hatched out of a very strong Irish Catholic tradition. Though I knew little of the social struggles of those earlier generations of Irish in Australia. I felt Australian in every way.

It was not until many years later when I wrote a verse novel, *Mostly Friday Nights*, about life in the suburbs in the seventies did I so fully realise how I had grown up in that particular bubble and that other people were raised under very different rules. For me, at that time, the Catholic way was absolute. There was an interplanetary gulf between us and the others in the town. At home, school and even in sport, I accepted the stern rule of authority as natural. Those in authority justified their power in that they were there to help us make something of ourselves in our future life. But their exercise of that power was not always fair.

One small example of how, as a young person, often in a state of fear, I lived far more in my head than in the physical world comes from when I was, again, in Second Grade at Saint John the Evangelist Primary School in Campbelltown. It was in the last week of year, just before we take the long Christmas break, and after we had done our end of year exams. I received the top mark in the class (495 out of 500). Each of us was asked to take our exam papers home to show our parents and then bring them back signed the next day, the penultimate day of the school year.

I dutifully took my paper home to show my parents who expressed due satisfaction with the result and signed the paper as requested. However, I failed to take the paper back to school the next day. I couldn't find it, even after searching everywhere in the house. As the teacher went along the rows to collect the papers from each of the students, I mustered the courage to say I forgot to bring it. My teacher advised me to hand it in the following day or I would not be able to proceed to Third Grade.

I was paralysed with fear. I frantically searched the house up and down again that night but couldn't find it. I went back to school the next day with my mind weighed down with this disaster as if I had committed a cardinal sin. I stayed quiet and didn't raise it with my teacher. After all, she was busy with other things on the last day of the school year.

But over that holiday break, all of December and January, I worried and worried that I would be made to repeat Second Grade because I hadn't done what the teacher had told me to do. The relief only came on that first day of school the following year when we all made our way to the room for Third Grade students and it seemed that the teacher had forgotten about the threat she made to me on that second last day of school. I had survived! So yes, I admit as a young person I was highly impressionable and was tangled in more mental and emotional worlds than the physical world itself. And I did find the paper a few years later. It had slipped down between a cupboard and the stove to gather dust.

Another example, some years later, of how I blindly accepted authority was at the minor event of registration day for the Under 12 cricket team. We assembled at the cricket oval in Hurley Park, a short walk from my home. We were young and having fun, thinking about the new season, about being involved in a team sport, with all my school friends wanting to be in the team. And I loved cricket because I had played so much in the backyard, at the oval and in the nets with friends, far from competition cricket. This day, we had cricket bags, filled with bats and balls, gloves and leg pads. I was excited, and we were horsing around with these new toys, and probably shouting a bit too much for those who were trying to organise us. We were asked to quieten down. Several times.

My exuberance got too much for one of the organisers, a son of one of the managers, one who fancied himself as both a cricketer and a coach. He stopped what he was doing and shouted at me. 'McGowan. I've had enough of you. Piss off home and never come back.'

I stopped and looked at him.

'You heard what I said. Go home. And stay home.'

I took him at his word. I walked away from that registration day and played no part in competition cricket for another three years. Young and in that environment, many of us lived too much inside our head. I didn't discuss it with anyone nor did I entertain the idea of appealing or challenging the judgement. I didn't dare seek the intervention of a higher authority.

It was only three years later and the Under 15s were starting the new season that I went along again and the new coach was a father of one of my classmates who loved cricket and believed in the life skills cricket had to offer. I went on to be one of the stock left arm off-spin bowlers. We won the competition that year. The best figures I got were 7-24 which even got me a mention in the local paper. Under my new coach's guidance I played district games for a season. It's also worth a note that in the eternal debate between the use of pace to remove a batsmen, to blast him out, versus the clever use of spin to bamboozle the batsmen, I was definitely on the side of 'use mind and not force'.

I do believe in the phenomenon of our attracting to ourselves evidence which supports our beliefs. So it made sense to me that when I opened the astrology pages of a magazine and read about Pisces, the author suggested that Pisces will lack confidence and be a bit otherworldly. That just confirmed it. But somewhere deep inside me there was an accumulated asking for more confidence and more worldliness.

As the seventies unfolded, authority was facing challenges from all directions. Even as the injuries and side effects of the Second World War were still washing through the system, the Cold War meant that world powers were locked into uncomfortable ideological positions which suggested a nuclear holocaust was not many shows of bravado away. Of course, these battles were being fought too far away for us to be meaningful players. But new movements sought to link local and global.

Meanwhile, unions and management struggled for shares of what was considered a pie of fixed size. Freedom was being shouted from high places, we faced social and political instability, censorship was being challenged, we had challenges to artistic, medical, scientific and educational norms. But to me, it was all way out there, somewhere else. I was in a comfortable school environment, busy with survival and wanting to be happy which largely consisted in keeping our parents, teachers and coaches happy, even as occasional shards of light from the outside world glinted in our eyes.

3 Early philosophy

My first introduction to philosophy was via my Uncle, Peter Carroll, my mother's older brother. Peter was a council worker for many years. He worked to earn enough money to live on. But he lived a rich inner life at home with his wife, Camille. Peter was a strict Catholic, and a Marxist. He would always say that both of the these systems of thought had the love of humanity at their core. He was an angry Marxist, an active trade unionist, one not afraid to stand up at union meetings and ask the uncomfortable questions, point his finger and lecture the leaders on the platform on the injustices of the capitalist system. And Peter was well read so if you wanted to argue with him you had better be ready. Peter turned his hand to so many things. I would visit his house on the weekend and he may be repairing his car, or building a veranda, or repairing a TV or radio or playing the harmonica, or listening to classical music. Or he could be reading books on science, theology, military history, or philosophy.

Peter spent his formative years in Manchester. He was bitter that he was thrown out of school as soon as he was capable of working a machine in a factory, hence his socialist leanings. It was Peter who patiently explained to me the movement of the working class intelligentsia, those men who engaged in menial work and who patiently educated and raised the political awareness of the many working men around them who essentially lived lives of despair.

It was Peter who told me that though he railed at the injustices of the system, his most passionate interest was in the field of metaphysics. He told me how he would lay awake at night and think and ask himself: 'Why am I here? What is this life all about?' I do believe that rather than simply influence me to be interested in metaphysics, it was something we shared, perhaps through family experience, or as an outcome of our religious upbringing. I do know that the field of metaphysics attracted me a lot more than political philosophy.

It was many years later, in my first year anthropology studies at university, when I sat up in some of the kinship classes where the lecturer pointed out that in many indigenous societies the mother's brother was one of the most important influences in a child's life. I have to admit that, in my case, I thought we may have stumbled on something more universal as I pondered on Peter's strong influence in my formative teenage years, away from both home and school. Regardless, I was lucky to spend time with someone so passionate and so curious about the world.

Even as my formative years were filled with getting an education which would set me up for a better life in the future, as well as working over the holidays, I also enjoyed playing football, cricket, some athletics and swimming, sports which allowed for the development of a range of skills, both individual and team.

I played the Rugby League code of football, a direct sport of people running into each other head on and trying to break through while the defensive team is trying to break their progress through tackling. Over 80% of the game is one dimensional ie moving forwards and backwards. When I got older, for some years, I played the Rugby Union code, a less direct football game where they work the ball around more an apply more strategy. I do recall how we could play on a Saturday afternoon and then have a shower and go out on Saturday night feeling okay whereas Rugby League would leave me feeling more battered and in need of rest. I have argued with a number of people who have different opinions about the effects of these two codes but this was my distinct experience.

While in primary school, my older sister and I were in awe of a guy in high school who lived down the street and had a black belt in karate. We tried to badger him into beating up a guy who was giving us trouble on our walks home from school. The black belt was a patient listener. He asked a lot of questions about who the trouble maker was and what the culprit had done before he told us to leave it with him. He was like our local strong man who meted out justice in the neighborhood as necessary.

Having played football, I felt I could benefit from some martial arts training to build myself up physically. But the right opportunity never presented itself to me. I went to one judo class with a friend in the Girl Guide's Hall in Hurley Park, a short walk from my house, but the teacher just ignored us and got a student to give us the introduction and that didn't seem to work for me. I never went back.

When I consider how my interest in martial arts grew, I still recall the TV series in the sixties called The Samurai, whose protagonist was Shintoro and his faithful servant was Tombei the Mist. It was exotic, it was about heroism, good versus evil, mystery and subterfuge, medieval romance, it was a break from the American westerns which didn't resonate so much with me at that time. When Shintoro and the Samurai team came to Australia in 1965 they saw a bigger crowd than that which welcomed the Beatles. I was fortunate enough to see them at the Sydney Stadium. I was sitting in a row behind which was a wide aisle and as Tombei the Mist ran past on his way to the stage he gently slapped my face. I felt special about that. This TV series captured our imagination. We would go off and play ninjas in the local park which had underground pipes and a drained dam overgrown with bullrushes up to two metres high. I didn't realise at that time how there were many who resented this importation of Japanese culture so soon after the Second World War and what was an Asian tradition and one that strayed from our own Judaeo-Christian traditions. But after all, Australia was a lot closer to Asia than Europe or the United States as we were to one day discover. In the last episode of season ten Shintoro disappeared from his group, last seen sailing off in the distance and that was the end of The Samurai. It was followed up by a new series, The Phantom Agents, set in a far more high tech environment, but with a lot of the same good versus evil themes in terms of martial artists defending both the greater good and the down-trodden individuals.

In my last years of high school, we were swept away by a new TV series out of the USA. It was Kung Fu and starred David Carradine as Kwai Chang Caine. The martial arts supremo, Bruce Lee was considered for the main role, but he was overlooked for a person of more mixed look as part of its desired audience appeal. Bruce Lee was indeed a fighting master, but so intense. Kwai Chang Caine was a lot more relaxed, more philosophical and part of the mythologised Shaolin tradition. This had to be the first time that the words of Lao Zi, the Chinese naturalist philosopher from centuries before Christ were ever recited on mainstream TV. Whatever we were doing, whatever our homework may be, we had to be ready on Tuesday nights for each of the new episodes of this show.

When I was 18, I went to a taekwondo class held at Wollongong University, and we were paired up for sparring. The fellow I was with was merciless. I thought he wanted to put me in hospital. I lasted one class. Again, I didn't see it as a way forward.

All these experiences led to a build up of wanting to know more and to live more of what seemed to be this long and powerful tradition. What resonated with me was that sense of development of a personal power which gave us a control over our lives even if we lived in the company of people who didn't share our values. We also accepted that a lot that life had to offer was out of reach. Implied in that was a sense it was time to get ready, keep your eye out for the opportunity and one day it would come.

In my final year of high school, I had no idea of what career would suit me. I'd read lots of career advisory information throughout the year but it was all a choppy sea of opportunity, a great expanse of unknown, into which I felt I was expected to dive and choose a career where I would discover new things, acquire new skills, but most importantly just get a job. It was a given that I would go to university as I had done well all through high school. The only advice my father gave to me was to study something and become good at it. He told me that, as a salesman who was pushed to chase bonuses and commissions for most of his life, he had constantly made a living off his wits and he always wished he had a profession.

But it was all so abstract. Most university subjects looked much the same to me on paper. Because I had such a good entry mark, I was blessed with so many options so I decided to just pick one and go with it. I eventually chose metallurgy and I won a metallurgy cadetship with Australian Iron and Steel in Port Kembla. This meant I would work four days and attend lectures one day and one evening each week, earning a wage while my employer put me through university. I was attracted to metallurgy for its simple definition of being a study of the science of metals. I saw the romantic side of this, a study of gold and silver and other precious metals. I know how to dream. But the reality was that, of course, being employed by the steelworks, it was simply training to make iron and steel.

4 The Kiama Bends

I was seventeen when I left home, setting out to work as a cadet metallurgist at the Port Kembla Steelworks run by Australian Iron and Steel. Six years of part-time study would see me become a Bachelor of Metallurgy. I took up a new residence in a new town, a new job, new study, and a new circle of friends. A lot of change. Before the year was out, my past and future collided in one of the most dramatic events in my life up until that time. This experience was part of my larger taiji journey.

On 13 September 1977 I crashed my car. I was the driver, still on learner plates. It occurred on a stretch of road called the Kiama Bends, a twisting road south of Kiama, a town on the NSW South Coast. My mate, Hughesy, was a passenger. The car was a cream Volkswagon beetle, an early sixties model, old and rusted, that I had bought cheap some months before. It happened as I was on my way to work, due to start at 9am.

Immediately before impact, I recall the car spinning out of control as if a hand from nowhere had lifted the back wheels off the road and the steering wheel no longer worked. It had been raining that morning and the road was slippery. I wasn't driving fast. I got to the crest of a rise and the road curved left. The car drifted to the right, and I tried to correct. I have since been told that the rear axle in those old V-Dubs had a design problem. But I now accept the cause of the accident was my lack of experience in handling the conditions.

The car was spinning round and round in circles no matter what I tried to do. I remember the road ahead was straight and the car was doing well at keeping to the centre of the road as it spun. Along this short stretch, we had a rock face on the left and a deep cliff behind a low safety fence on the right. The car chose to spin into the rock face. Slam! The car crunched into the rock; the sound of metal, the final clunk of the motor, and a long silence. That silence of the lonely windswept road overlooking a deep fall down to the steely white-tipped sea was only broken by that of dripping fluid which I immediately thought was petrol.

Hughesy had been asleep in the back seat of the car at the moment of impact. Now he was laying against the firewall in the front. I can't remember seeing him flung there. My seat was rusted where it was bolted to the floor. The impact of the prang ripped the seat off the floor. My face hit the windscreen, with my mouth catching the steering wheel on the way through. It hit hard enough to knock a top front tooth out. But I was alive. And conscious.

Thinking about the possibility of a fuel leak in the front of the car, I was panicked into action. I opened my door and dragged Hughesy from the car. I sat him down about ten metres away from the car. I was feeling very light headed by that time. I hadn't paused to assess the pain that was burning both my face and legs.

The next sequence is dream-like. I heard a car approaching from the same direction we had come. Standing near Hughesy, I waved my arms in the air and I saw faces in the front and back seat of the car just staring open-mouthed as their car sped by. I put my hand to face and realised that it was covered in blood. To be fair they couldn't see the damaged section of the car pressed into the rock face so all they could see was a parked car and two guys, one sitting and one standing, the standing guy with a bloody face. They may have assessed it as too dangerous to stop.

More aware of the stinging pain across every inch of my face, I sat down and began some breathing exercises for pain control. Around that time, I was keenly interested in a book called *Relief Without Drugs* written by a Melbourne doctor Ainslie Meares. Such books are all too common today but at that time it was a pioneer text. He actually had exercises in the book where you stuck pins in your arm and you practised to detach from the pain. Out here, I likewise looked at my pain while I remained detached. It worked. So there was Hughesy now sprawled out on the ground and me and the car smashed against the side of the road on that damp grey south coast morning.

A short while later, another car stopped and a lady walked up to us, a short warrior type of lady, very confident. She asked: "What's happened, boys?"

We gawked at her silently.

She next asked where we were from.

"Campbelltown," I replied, still gathering my thoughts to tell her what had happened.

"Me too," she cut in. So one of our own came to help us. She went to look at Hughesy. Other people arrived on the scene. Their bodies were close but their voices were far away. I think they were looking at the car.

The Campbelltown lady was leaning close to Hughesy. He was babbling on, using lots of words to say that he didn't know what had happened. This was surprising for me because Hughesy was one of the coolest people I ever knew and he had been through some testing moments in his life and he always seemed to know what to say and what to do. But he just kept on going around in circles saying things like, 'Well, ah, funny you should ask that. Uh, because, actually, you see, I just can't remember what happened. Don't you think that's crazy?' All in his confident, gunfire manner.

Meanwhile, the lady came over to me. I told her I had swallowed glass. She, in turn, told the ambulance driver who had since arrived. So they slowly placed us in the back of the ambulance. Once I was resting in there, I remember one of the officers leaning over me and saying: 'I'll use this pump to get the glass out.' And he kept fiddling with the equipment next to him just out of my range of sight. A stomach pump I believe. But he was taking so long.

He mumbled something to himself and then he turned to me. 'Sorry, mate, but I can't get it to work. We have to wait until we get back to the hospital.' I was still thinking about how I'd be late for work.

The other thing I remember about the ride to the hospital was the strong sense of reassurance the heavy suspension of an ambulance van instils within you. This felt good as my mind drifted to the outer orbits. I also remember Hughesy's chatter with the driver about how he couldn't remember who was driving. I later found out that ambulance drivers are responsible for making one accident report and then the police conduct an interview later to make a second report.

So we get to the hospital. I am lying on a table and I hear the nurse telling others she can smell alcohol.

'You fellows haven't been drinking have you?' Her voice had the tone of a schoolmistress.

"No," I replied, innocently. They discovered I had some barley sugar lollies in my pocket and she reluctantly accepted she was wrong. I still don't know if they did a blood alcohol test.

I was told I would need a full set of x-rays urgently. So two nurses brutally press my face into the table and the pain of the glass in my face increased a hundredfold. Then I was rolled around for the next x-ray so that only half of my face was pressed against the table this time. And then the other side. I began to feel like I was on a chopping block. All this time, Hughesy was sitting behind a curtain talking with doctors and nurses. He had gone beyond his claimed loss of memory and was telling them how to contact his family. Meanwhile I drifted into sleep.

At that time, I was living at Weerona, a hostel for Port Kembla Steelworks trainees and apprentices. That semester I went to university every Tuesday. Hughesy lived back in Campbelltown with his parents. Hughesy mixed the sound for a band called *Da Syndicate* which played in Kings Cross on weekends. It was school holidays at the time and two girls we knew were caravanning down the South Coast with their families.

Many things went wrong in a short period of time. There were many warning signs I failed to read. I ignored these signs as I pushed on, preferring a forced path over one of more mindful steps. Hughesy drove me down to Wollongong the Sunday night before. It was my car, but as I had no licence, only a learner's permit, I left the car with Hughesy during the week. The car broke down on Bulli Pass, ten kilometres north of Wollongong. We parked the car at the bottom of the Pass and walked back to Wollongong. A colleague at the hostel, was dabbling with tarot cards at that time. When we got back, he spread the cards for us and he was shocked at how bad they looked, to the point where he didn't want to go on. All the dark scary cards were there. But we didn't lose much sleep over it. Hughesy went the next day to get the car repaired. It needed a new accelerator cable. And I went off to work as I did every Monday.

Our plan was to go down the coast to see our friends on Tuesday instead of me going to University. It was over two hours by car. So

Hughesy arrived early and we headed off after breakfast. We went to the caravan park at Lake Tabourie as arranged and couldn't find the girls anywhere. Couldn't find them, their family car or their caravan! And so we went to all the other caravan parks in the area looking for them. And we couldn't contact them by phone. So we spent most of the day searching. Out of luck, we headed home. Not long after getting back at dinner time, one of the friends called us. She wanted to know where we were. She gave us an exact description of where to find her. So we made a snap decision to head back down there, and spend a few hours together that night. I would go straight to work from there the next morning.

By the time we arrived it was already late, long gone dark. But we met as planned and just all four of us sat in the car and talked and joked and smoked cigarettes for a few hours. My friend's parents were expecting them back around ten so eventually they had to go. Driving now was out of the question. So we decided to get some sleep in the car right where it was parked. The nights are still cool in September. But we got a few hours sleep so that I had lots of time to get to work that next morning.

It was a grey, overcast south coast morning. As we moved up the coast, it was obvious they'd had some rain during the night. I remember getting out of the car when we stopped to buy petrol and thinking how the weather was not going to get much better that day. I also remember the guy who pumped our petrol. He didn't say a word. He probably just had the early morning blues, though I wondered later whether his sullen manner was some sort of warning to us. Anyhow Hughesy said he was tired and offered me to drive.

'Yeah, Why not? There's no traffic,' I said.

So Hughesy lay in the back seat to nap. I was content to drive at an easy speed and just patiently move through the morning to something better.

Then it happened.

Later that morning, Hughesy's father, a welfare worker at Campbelltown Court, was sitting in a court room when he received the message about his son. He was sitting next to a cop from the South Coast at the time. He told him what had happened. The cop took the note off Charlie and pulled out a pen and wrote down a name and a telephone number, saying: 'I suggest you talk to my colleague.'

That call to the police friend helped in many ways: 'Before you go any further, let me tell you what he had in his boot. He had a small TV, a stereo radio/cassette player and.......they enjoy traveling and always take a lot of stuff with them where ever they go." The cop was relieved because upon first seeing the contents of the boot, they thought they had caught members of a burglary ring.

A few days later, when another policeman visited me in hospital, he took out his notebook, asked a few questions, made some notes and quietly left. So there I was in the hospital bed, with a battered unrecognisable face, full of stitches across the nose, eyelid, cheeks and lips, a front tooth missing and a banged up knee. I felt abandoned, though little did I know at the time that the students at daily assembly at my old school were being asked to keep me in their prayers. The hospital had a practice of clearing beds on Friday to make way for new intakes expected over the weekend. And this was in 1977! So Dad came to collect me on Friday afternoon.

I still remember standing in the lounge room at home when a few friends came around to visit. One good friend, Ozzie, was a very relaxed person. I still remember the look of shock on his face when he first saw my stitched up face. I could barely talk and was on a liquid diet because I couldn't open my mouth very wide.

The next Sunday when Dad drove me to church for evening mass, he stopped the car in a parking space close to church. I can't remember any desire to offer a prayer of thanks for being alive. It's just what we used to do each week.

Looking straight ahead, he began: 'When your mother was cleaning your clothes she found some marijuana in your jacket.'

He was still talking but I recalled that neat new jacket I wore when we went to pubs and discos. One of the jacket pockets had a hole in it. One day I pushed a glad bag of dope through the hole and worked it to the back of the jacket. I thought this was brilliant. I could hide anything in an instant. I must have forgot about it. There was little chance of anyone finding it. But Mum did.

He continued: 'If I was your age I would probably be smoking too.' He turned to me. 'But what you need to remember is that this is a dirty business and people just sell it to make money and they don't care what they sell you and whether it's good for you or not.' That reminded me of the bomb VW I had bought. 'So you ought to think about whether you should be smoking the stuff or not.'

I was going: 'Yeah, yeah.' I couldn't think of anything to say, all I was thinking was that Dad had picked his words so well and was good at getting his message across. He was an experienced salesman after all. He wasn't wasting his words.

The months went by, and as Hughesy's father predicted I was still picking glass from my face. I went back to work and study and got my replacement tooth.

Technically, I was on the way to work the morning of the crash so I was entitled to worker's compensation which was duly paid. I was never asked questions about whether I attended university the day before, or what in the hell was I doing coming to work via Kiama. And I don't know if any of my colleagues were asked, but the bureaucratic machine rolled right on past these questions.

My new obsession was putting on seatbelts before my car ever started. That habit continues through to the present day. This however needs to be weighed against my overwhelming belief that I was meant to be alive. It was at about this time that I developed my idea of self-insurance. I joked with others that I had no need to take out comprehensive insurance because there were only two possibilities: one was that because I followed the road rules so closely and I had been so well trained in driving the idiot's car, that most likely the other party would be at fault if I was in any prang. And if I was at fault then most likely it would be such a bad accident that I would probably be killed.

Something unusual happened at the same spot ten years later. My family had since moved to Berry, about half an hour by car past Kiama. And I was working at a health food store and clinic in Rozelle. Some weekends, I would make the trip to Berry after finishing work late on a Saturday afternoon. It was one Saturday evening when I was flagged down by an elderly man telling me to slow down as there was a crash up ahead. I pulled over behind the queue of cars. I wasn't keen to get involved because I had only little experience in emergency situations. Two or three other drivers were busy tending some people on the side of the road. One man was throwing dirt onto the exposed motor of the crashed car. To stop it from igniting I guessed. The driver must have been speeding because the front of the car was badly damaged.

I walked closer to the car in question and saw the driver inside. His legs were trapped under the steering wheel, his feet were pinned under the pedals on the floor and his door couldn't open. As the rescuers focused on other family members and the car itself, I just walked up and opened the front passenger's door and got in. I sat next to the guy pinned there. His eyes were strained with fear.

'Easy mate,' I said, 'your wife and kids are okay.'

I knew where he was at. He was half stuck in the unknown and afraid of it, and half floating free of it and unsure.

'Look, the best thing you can do is just settle. Feel your breath, mate.' I was teaching taiji and meditation in classes back in Sydney. And I knew the enormous value of meditation. So I just kept talking calmly.

'Watch your breath. Feel it as you inhale. Feel it as you exhale.' He was responding. He was letting go. So I kept on reassuring him. *Reassure the patient*, I forget where I had heard this catchcry, but I was dismayed that this guy had been so ignored by the others at the crash scene.

I said, 'Mate, they'll get you out of here. Take you to hospital to check everything. And then you can go home to rest. With your family.' His eyes reacted as if to say 'thank you,' that he appreciated the assistance, however small.

'Where do you work?' I asked. 'The steelworks. Engine driver.'

My head went 'Bing'! I casually replied, 'Interesting. I worked there ten years ago. And you know I had a prang right here on this same spot. See these scars.' I said pointing to scars on cheek and nose. He tried to look just as I had asked him.

'The best thing you can do for now is calm yourself. And time will heal all,' I repeated.

Some boisterous guy dressed in overalls swaggered up and stuck his head in the car window and shouted, 'So here's our patient! No worries, mate, we'll have you out of here in no time.' He signalled to his colleague carrying a chain saw. 'This door has to come off. Let's get started.'

'I better move on,' I said quietly, 'so good luck.' I went back to my car. The traffic now had a way through the accident scene. I cruised past the damaged car unable to see into it, just listening to the chain saw biting the door. I looked forward, on to my destination.

As I saw my crash from a different perspective, I wondered how this man's life would change in coming months and years as I realised just how much my experience heralded so much change in my inner life which would soon enough manifest into my outer life.

5 Getting closer

Despite the loudness of the message I had just received, the steps to any new life were small at first, mostly restricted to my inner world, nothing more than the occasional spark of a new thought, idea or impulse. But they slowly got louder. I was not always a willing participant in this change process. Even as the new beckoned me, I felt like I was still in a wash cycle not knowing when it would end. As I sought to keep my work and study routines on track, I found relief from inner anxiety with an above average share of drinking, smoking and party-going.

I worked my critical eye hard, turning cynicism into a high art. I felt like I alone could see through the frayed veil of many of our social conventions. But I had little idea what to do about it. A good example of how my rampant doubts clashed head on with my life was my take on science. Here I was studying science at university and yet I could not accept the claim that scientists were neutral and objective in their practice as they claimed. I saw them as avid believers in their holy activity, many with a burning passion for their work. They were anything but the dispassionate observers they professed to be. For me, it was religion all over again. Science was a club where its members dealt with threats to their elevated importance, be they from inside or outside, by turning on those who threatened them by labelling them as either unscientific or pseudo-scientific. I was becoming a member of a club I found it hard to believe in.

Science at this time was making a lot more promises than delivering results. But the revolution was on the way. This was the late seventies and very few in Australia were working in the computer field. In first year chemistry, our lecturer, at the start of the year boldly stated that the future was in computers and we should work to gain as much exposure to computers and computing as we could. At that time, we were only enrolled in Fortran programming and the resources for students were extremely limited (finding a free terminal to key in your program) so that it was easier to share your exercises with class colleagues. We weren't so concerned about the future. We just wanted to pass our subjects.

I couldn't complain about my metallurgy course. It's just that my heart wasn't in it. In fact, my abiding memory is of some outstanding lecturers. One was Nick Standish who lectured on thermodynamics. One day he explained how he awarded full marks to one student who was asked to write a one page essay on the second law of thermodynamics and that student simply wrote the words: 'Water flows downhill'. Nick thought this was the perfect answer. Extra words would just cloud any explanation! We were also impressed by Professor Noel Kennon who lectured in crystallography. He was like a doctor in diagnosing crystal structures. He had a flair for analysing a slice of failed metal under a microscope and being able to give the history of the metal and the reason for its failure. He was the go-to man for difficult cases from the Steelworks.

I remember sitting in the classroom listening to lectures on thermodynamics and crystallography etc and looking out the window with my ears ringing, I wanted to be somewhere else, doing something else. When I shared these thoughts with my friends and family, how I was so tired of this study, they urged me to continue, that it would only be another three or four years. I, in turn, began to feel the pressure of wasting precious time.

Another small step forward, one great source of relief, for me during those study years was my daily practice of a kung fu exercise routine I had begun at home. I found it in a book called *The Kung Fu Exercise Book: Health Secrets of Ancient China* written by Michael Minick and described as silk-weaving exercises.

These were essentially 14 Shaolin exercises to strengthen the body and mind. Michael put the exercises within the broader context of the Asian martial arts tradition and he explained their close relationship with Chinese medicine which had been practised for fifty centuries. Through this book, in a very simple way, he communicated the theory of Chinese medicine to many Westerners for the very first time. For him the essential contrast between Western and Chinese medicine was that health in Western medicine was based on a defence against invasion from external threats, whereas Chinese medicine was more about generating health through the strengthening of our internal organs.

The Kung Fu Exercise Book: Health Secrets of Ancient China is a book with a lot of white space. Michael, I am sure, set out to engage the reader without overloading them with information. He knew that his book was but a door to a much larger world, so all he had to do was spark the interest in the reader, and help them through that door.

As soon as I picked this book up in the shop, I knew it was something for me. This happens from time to time and feels so good when it does. I continued to do those exercises every morning for the next two years. I didn't really know it at that time, but this was the perfect preparation for my eventual introduction to taiji. The exercises were still physical, with some reference to breathing and meditation, but they were enough. Minick does mention deep in the book that it won't work to run out and find a teacher but rather a teacher will come to the reader when the time is right. I accepted his word on that.

My hunger for what may be best described as hidden knowledge continued to grow. I read books on all sorts of occult subjects including astrology, tarot, numerology, palmistry and mysticism in general. The reader may be able to see why my hostility to science was so strong. I recall reading a novel by Aleister Crowley and getting interested in his ideas. The University of Wollongong Library held a few of his books which I pored over, understanding very little except that it was way out there. This was only heightened by the knowledge that members of my favourite band, Led Zeppelin, also had strong interest in the works of Crowley. I also marveled at the works of the palm reader Cheiro and how he travelled the world meeting wealth and royalty with his skills of reading character and fortune in the palm of the hand. I sensed that science as taught at school and university didn't have a monopoly on truth.

A year after I started the silk-weaving exercises, I also started a very simple daily meditation routine. This was inspired by *Three Magic Words,* a work by novelist and new age writer, Uell Stanley Anderson. In this book he began by describing his search for spiritual understanding and went on to share the answers he had received. I suppose I was wanting some answers badly. He provided a detailed account of what he calls 'the infinite mind' which pervades all things. His observation was that most of us forget the nature and power of this infinite mind and we tend to get swayed by what we may call 'the momentary mind'.

So Uell's mission was to remind people of the infinite mind and to help them to connect it up to the momentary mind.

What was good about this book, as in the kung fu book, was that the author advised a program of 10 to 15 minutes of meditation per day followed by a reading of a paragraph of affirmations at the end of each chapter. I was taken in by this book because it was so sweeping in its sources, everything form Plato to Christ to Nietzsche, I kept it by my bedside for well over a year. It was a lifeline for me as I broke from the cocoon of my upbringing to become a person more able to enjoy and appreciate and engage with this amazing world around me.

I looked for group activities to become involved in and with my housemate, I joined the local branch of the Friends of the Earth (FOE) a group founded by US conservationist David Brower. It was a small group, we were led by two very committed local high school teachers. Our biggest involvement was helping to set up and run a stall at an Energy Fair held in 1978 at an oval in Oak Flats, south of Wollongong.

By 1979, my car crash was a distant memory. But the changes emanating from it continued. It simply made sense to look around for other career opportunities. By enrolling in metallurgy, I felt like I had dived too quickly into a specialist field of study. I decided it would have been better to study something more general and work my way into a more specialised area. I would recommend to anyone in high school who is not sure of exactly what they are wanting to do, to try something general to begin with and they can later zoom in on whatever special area attracts them.

Also, I had long wanted to live in Sydney. So I planned to study at Sydney University and try something new. I applied to enrol in an arts degree. In discussing this decision with my Uncle Peter, his advice, given the cerebral focus, was for me to do something with my hands to keep a good balance. I decided I would take my silk-weaving exercises to a new level and take up a martial art.

I was discussing this with a friend at the Steelworks in the section where I was still working. He held a black belt in karate. He told me that there were many styles of martial arts. He said that taiji was the most powerful but it took the longest to learn. He explained that it was more to do with the mind and how it directed the energy rather than using brute force. Not a bad summation of the art.

Another moment in my emerging awareness of taiji was my watching Francis Ford Coppola's film *Apocalypse Now* where Martin Sheen, in the role of Captain Benjamin Willard, on a journey up the Mekong River, did taiji on the deck of their small river boat each morning. Willard's journey was a metaphor for a journey through the psyche of the modern American mind, in the same vein as Dante's journey through the levels of hell in *Inferno*. The film captured that dual function of taiji, and how we play the roles of both spectator and player in life.

I was in no hurry to start but I decided to explore taiji. I wasn't consciously aware of the momentum I had generated with my interest in the kung fu silk weaving exercises, and my dabbling in philosophy which had been inspired by the *Kung Fu* TV series. It felt like an impulse but only a mild type of impulse. I do think now that I was being guided by my inner being, but I had to be receptive. To move from the secure path of metallurgist with guaranteed employment to a general arts degree with an unknown future was a big statement that personal wellbeing was of greatest importance to me at that time. As it turned out, there was an economic downturn in the early eighties and many of metallurgist and chemical engineer colleagues received redundancies. A lot of automation was being introduced to the Steelworks in those years. I sometimes joke that I was simply ahead of the curve with my career move.

Reflecting on the above events, I can almost see a script, but for me on the ground, I felt little direction. There was no joining of the dots and there were very few 'Hell! Yes!' moments. Even my decision to seek out a taiji class felt okay but I can't say it was powerful. It just felt right. But that evening I walked into my first taiji class, I felt an overwhelming 'Hell!Yes!' This was something I had wanted for a long time.

6 Introduction to taiji

I celebrated my twenty-first birthday on a Saturday night at my parents' home. The next morning, I set out for the big smoke of Sydney with all my worldly possessions in the boot and back seat of my HR Holden. There was much organising to do, like find a place to live and be ready for lectures in two day's time. I was helped by a school friend who had a house in Stanmore, one suburb from Sydney Uni. He put me up for a week before I found a room in a share house close by.

I made it to my first taiji class the following Tuesday night. In seeking this class, I wasn't shopping for a teacher or a style. I found the class via a huge bundle of student information I received when I enrolled. It was held in the Sydney University Women's Gym administered by Sydney University Women's Sports Association (founded in 1910). I could see a certain resonance that taiji, an art that preaches strength through softness, would gravitate towards the Women's Gym. In 2003, the Sydney University Women's Sports Association merged with the Sydney University Sports Union to form Sydney Uni Sport and Fitness.

The class was in a huge hall. Early in the term, the numbers were big, almost thirty students, filling a large part of the space. As the weeks wore on, students dropped out. Perhaps they wanted something more vigorous or they had found what they wanted, had their questions answered, or were just too busy as they narrowed down their long list of extra-curricular interests.

For me, attending this class was like a rendezvous. It was total validation of my decision to relocate to Sydney and start all over again. Simon Lim, the teacher, was a short man, an Indonesian Chinese who wore a colourful batik shirt. My first impression of him was that he stamped absolute authority on his class with his booming voice. He spoke clearly, concisely, yet with a balance of gentle and firm. One got the immediate impression that Simon was the newest generation of a long line of taiji teachers who went back centuries. His knowledge and his expression of that knowledge was so full and yet so immediately useful to all of us.

Each of us in the room felt like Simon was standing in front of us individually, talking to us one-on-one, knowing where we were at and answering all of our questions.

The introduction to taiji was deceptively simple. I had previously been told that taiji took the longest amount of time to learn. In fact, Simon taught his senior students a long form of 128 postures. But his introductory classes focused on a basic set of five flowing exercises. The theory of traditional Chinese medicine is based on the interaction of five primary elements. Each of these elements has a series of fundamental correspondences. And so it was with taiji, we had the five flowing exercises. These were:

1. Hand Play with clouds: metal element, governing lungs and large intestines, movement left and right;
2. Brushing the knee, water elements, governing kidney and water bladder, movement forwards;
3. Repulse the monkey, wood element, governing liver and gall bladder, movement backwards;
4. Crane Opens wings: fire element, governing heart and small intestine, movement up and down;
5. Brush Swallow's Tail: earth element, governing spleen and stomach, movement all round.

By mastering these exercises we had a self contained exercise routine that we could practise at home and even teach another person. By doing each exercise for five minutes, plus some standing meditation at the start and finish of the routine, it made up half an hour of a taiji routine.

At the beginning and end of each class, Simon had us stand quietly to do breathing meditation. I have never seen such a simple and powerful relaxation exercise. He would get us to let our breath come in, and then breathe out to the extremities of our body, out to our hands, to our feet and to the point at the top of our head. It was half based on imagining the flow of our breath even as we felt it. This was a practical introduction to how to flow our qi energy in our body, that thing we could not see, or touch or hear, but we could feel it. It was the essence of qi gong health exercise.

We often had our eyes closed as Simon took us through the exercise, to feel our feet touching the ground, feeling steady and stable, earthed, even if we were standing on the moon we would still be well-earthed. The point on the ball of our feet where we did touch the ground was a well-known acupuncture point called the bubbling springs. Feeling the top of our head at a point which Chinese medicine calls the bai hui, the hundred places meeting point. We also know it as the halo point. This helps us to lighten up, feel more awake, energise our brain. We also felt our hands more energised, thick and warm, as we prepare to do work, find a way to make use of menial tasks, we can express ourselves through our hands. So we had this idea that we can direct our energy to the extremities of our body, but in the future we would be able to direct energy to any part of our body that needed help. This was beneficial so that even as I earned money in my first few years at university picking up glasses and cleaning ashtrays at the local RSL Club, I enjoyed this work thinking I was using my time well by practising to breathe out through my hands as I worked. I could even still feel fresh at the end of my shift!

The first term of taiji classes was spent learning the five flowing exercises. In the following terms we were introduced to the longer form. During these early lessons, Simon spoke so much about just getting the whole body moving. He used the analogy of getting to see the whole forest before we go in to adjust the individual trees. What this meant with the longer form of taiji was that we would do it continuously. Simon would break down a few of the individual postures only once or twice at the end of the night. If we wanted to see them again, we had to wait until the following week. Some struggled to learn the form for this reason. They desperately wanted Simon to stop each posture so they could study it more closely, and then put all the postures back together again. Simon was of the idea that if you wanted to examine a living being you couldn't kill it and dissect it without actually destroying it. It's a bit like getting to know what's inside an egg without smashing the shell. So he urged students to just enjoy the flow of taiji postures over the hour and slowly the body will remember the postures.

By the end of the year I had remembered all 128 postures so that over the summer break, I was able to practise alone at home each day. And when I went on to teach taiji, I found it really interesting that some students would corner me and ask me to stop so they could understand the postures but it didn't seem to help very much. And this was one of the great lessons of studying taiji in a university environment: it is not something to be grasped intellectually. It was a total experience of mind, body and breath. And I understood this. In retrospect, I had been preparing for the taiji opportunity a long time before I ever walked into any class.

Simon was incredibly busy outside his main job of running a health food store. He taught taiji at both University of Sydney and University of NSW. He was also teaching prisoners at Long Bay Jail, and he ran his own school at the Uniting Church Hall in Canterbury. His school was like a wheels within wheels network. If people wanted to know what taiji was, learn some relaxation technique, or just do simple taiji exercises, introductory classes were widely available. But there was always the opportunity for those students more interested to dig deeper.

Having mastered the form in the first year, in the second and third years, I helped teach the form to students who had completed their introductory terms. Simon would run the introduction in one half of the auditorium while I went through the first two cycles at the other end of the hall. Mid-way through the class, he would take a break and dash over to us and take us all through the form and explain more of taiji, qi breathing and flowing the qi through our body. Even as Simon moved from one group to the other, by the end of the night, everyone was satisfied with what they were learning.

As a nominal senior student at the Sydney University Women's Gym, Simon encouraged me to go out to the classes he ran at Canterbury on Monday and Wednesday evenings. This was another level of taiji school. Few of the Sydney University students fed into this class. Simon had attracted the Canterbury students over a few years by word of mouth. At that time, the profile of your average taiji student was a person from the fringes, people interested in natural therapies, musicians, artists, unemployed, people sympathetic to new age ideals. Of course there were students with mainstream occupations, eg lab workers, lawyers, call centre operators, public servants and firemen, each with their own story to tell. It truly was a modern day rendition of Chaucer's *Canterbury Tales*.

Canterbury's Uniting Church Hall is an old stone hall on the very busy Canterbury Road. It was always a trek from the city whether by car or on the peak hour train service. It was a welcome shelter from the cold in the winter months and a place of shade in the summer months. The class went on and on week after week showing Simon's commitment to his students and the art.

Out here, Simon offered in-depth meditation training. His aim was that he wanted to teach teachers and so he spoke to a very high level of understanding of taiji with more about the history of the art.

Simon also welcomed students to his house in Campsie (by the railway line) on Saturday afternoons and Sunday mornings where he ran his natural health clinic from the front room of his house. He also trained students with supplementary taiji exercises of pushing body and pushing hands in the backyard. These were exercises that needed refinement and practice and there was never enough time in class to explore these aspects of taiji.

I had much momentum going to taiji classes 3 or 4 times a week as well as Simon's place on weekends. I was doing something I loved and I felt that there were so much to learn and absorb.

While I originally said that I enrolled at university to study philosophy and do taiji as something to occupy my hands, as each year progressed, I was giving taiji more and more of my focus and treating my uni study as the hobby.

It was a world of discovery, mixing with people with very progressive beliefs and we all knew that we had the best taiji teacher in Sydney, a guy who was really focussed on the essence of taiji in the most authentic way. The general taiji landscape in Sydney in the early eighties was that there were several big schools in Sydney: The largest was Gary Khor. There were also Tennyson Yu, Dean Rainer, and Erle Montague, all teachers with good names. But Simon was like a loner who stuck to a non-commercial and very person-based model of the art.

But taiji was so formless, outwardly here I was, studying an undergraduate degree at university, earning a living to support my study as I maintained my links with my family, even as I formed new friendships and set up home in a new city. There seemed to be so much change in such a short time, but the taiji idea was that change would always be occurring so we needed to learn how to best go along with it. I moved house about ten times in my four years of study at university. I always felt busy because my time was filled with learning more and more about taiji and natural healing.

7 The form

To do taiji is to consciously experience the full co-ordination of mind, body and breath. In this chapter, we will explore the phenomenon of the taiji form.

To the casual observer, the taiji form may appear as a series of self-defence postures. However, it is a cultural masterpiece of design compacted with an ever-unfolding series of information, revelations and guidance about the nature of who we really are as human beings. The names of the postures themselves often carry symbolic cultural references. The form holds valuable instruction relating to breathing exercises, meditation, philosophy, alchemy practice, and traditional systems of medicine and therapy. A person may learn taiji without being informed about these cultural transmissions, but if they were to continue with their taiji exercise each day, a time would come when these elements buried deep within the form will rise to the surface and reveal themselves.

Here I will would like to provide an example of the richness of the form. The first of the five flowing exercises taught to beginners is called Hand Play with the Clouds.

Firstly, when we perform taiji, we are shifting weight from one foot to the other constantly moving backwards and forwards, we are never double-weighted, and when there is tension in one foot there is an increased tension in the hand on the opposite side of the body. And likewise, when one foot is free of tension, let's say relaxed, the hand on the opposite side of the body feels less tension, is more relaxed than the other hand. Now when we draw a line from the tense foot to the tense hand and then another line from the relaxed foot to the relaxed hand, we see that they cross over in the centre of the body in the abdominal region. Our centre is both tense and relaxed.

The Hand Play with the Clouds flowing exercise demonstrates movement to the left and the right. As weight shifts from the left foot to the right foot and back as the arms move in circles, the left arm moving anti-clockwise and the right arm moving clockwise. As the left hand is at eye level ie the top of the anti-clockwise circle, the right hand is at waist level, ie the bottom of the clockwise circle, and vice-versa. As we experience the movement to both left and right, we better establish ourselves at the centre of the motion. We yield to the left and yield to the right to feel the full balance of the centre. This is all happening as we are nonstop shifting weight from one foot to the other. So at the physical level we are exercising every part of our body as we gently stretch and relax. This has a massaging effect on the organs in our body.

Apart from learning how we differentiate and integrate contrasting yin and yang movement to the left and the right, we have noted in the last chapter how this posture is allocated to the element of metal. In Chinese medicine theory, metal governs the lung function in the body, and the lungs partner with the large intestine. So this first flowing is a complete exercise in itself, it is traditionally seen as benefiting the lung and large intestine function in particular.

At another level, this flowing exercise becomes a meditation on the water cycle. With the circular motion of each of our hands, we follow the path water takes as it falls to the earth, evaporates up to the sky to form clouds which produce rain, and this rain again falls to the earth. An endless process.

This meditation on the water cycle in turn reinforces the physical action of the exercise. When the weight is on the right foot, the left hand is at its lowest point in the circle. Similarly, when the weight is on the left foot, the right hand is at the lowest point. Because there is more tension in each hand when it is at these lowest points compared to when it is at the top of their circles. The hand, as it passes through the cloud, feels lighter, more relaxed. And as it passes through the water, it feels heavier, with more tension. So the cloud-water imagery assists the physical expression of the taiji flowing.

There are many taiji forms. The particular form of a taiji school is simply the vehicle for transmission of taiji from teacher to student, though form is not the teacher's alone as it also carries their particular lineage. Form (Japanese martial artists call it kata) can be over-rated. A good teacher makes full use of their form at hand to communicate the taiji idea. A good student uses the available form to engage with the teacher and share their experience.

Now and then, you may get a form that resonates deeply with what a person is seeking. This was so with the form that I learned. It was the best form I could have possibly found, the way it aligned with the accompanying Chinese philosophy of nature.

First I want to locate taiji within the broader martial arts spectrum. In Chinese pugilistics, we have internal and external martial arts. The external martial arts, think of the Shaolin arts, are based on strengthening the bones, muscles and tendons. Speed and strength become key physical attributes and a highly disciplined mind is the key nonphysical attribute. Such training is detailed and extensive. Consider the martial artist exercise for strengthening the fingers, where the student holds a pot of sand and bangs their fingers into the sand hundreds and hundreds of times per session. To graduate from an external martial arts school is a test of physical and mental endurance.

We do have other martial arts described as internal. They profess a focus on energy flow in the body. Taiji, an evasive art based on the principles of water, and is known as the queen of the internal martial arts. Bagua, an explosive art based on the principles of fire, is known as the king of the internal arts. For a bagua fighter, a fight lasts only a matter of seconds. We also have another popular internal art called xingyi, a simple yet powerful form. Over the centuries, there have been numerous obscure spin-offs in the way people cultivate their internal energy. For example, there is one tradition of the well-fist where the student assumes the horse posture and points his fists at a nearby well and directs their energy towards it. After three years, the student is supposed to be able to make the water mildly turbulent and after ten years they will be able to kill an aggressor from a distance.

The proliferation of taiji forms is to be expected as we see the art taught all over China in many schools over many centuries. It is like the spread of languages across the world.

In 1956, the Peking All China Physical Training Society instigated a shortened taiji form of 24 postures as part of the national health program The goal was to make the health benefits of taiji more accessible to all citizens. The government did not necessarily want to produce taiji masters but it wanted its citizens to be healthy and productive members of society.

Today, when we look on Wikipedia, at the listing of taiji forms, we see over 80 forms. They range from routines with four moves all the way to routines with 229 moves. Curiously, the form of 128 postures that I learned was still not on that list at the time of writing this book. The form with 128 postures is particularly appealing because it suggests a direct relationship with the *Yi Jing*, an ancient Chinese work of philosophy.

As I will reference this work several times, at this point I will briefly introduce the Yi Jing, often translated as the Book of Change or the Classic of Changes. Said to have been written about 1000BC, it is described as a book of divination, but it is also a collection of sayings and ideas on history, culture, philosophy and cosmology. While being so ancient, it still serves as a guide to Chinese culture in many dimensions. Even recent speeches of current President of China, Xi Jin Ping, reference the work. For example, in 2018 he spoke of the need for people to 'tirelessly strengthen' themselves (zìqiángbùxī) which is directly lifted from the commentary of the first chapter of the *Yi Jing*.

In short, the *Yi Jing* consists of 64 chapters. The 'logic' of these chapters is built on the repeated division of one single unit into two, with 64 being one unit divided seven times. My taiji form contains 128 postures, a doubling of 64, or two raised to the power of seven. This form is very philosophical in its design and resonates with the profundity of the Yi Jing, but let's take one step at a time. Whatever form we do choose to practise, we must marvel at the distillation of human experience that goes into that form.

Very much in the spirit of that division and subdivision which the *Yi Jing* catalogues, the taiji forms as mentioned are many and varied. In summary, most accounts of taiji list the four major schools. Taiji was nurtured for many generations in a Chen family village in Henan Province. They subdivided into the new and old Chen forms with the new Chen form being called Yang. As these forms interacted, the Wu style was developed. Much later, at the start of the twentieth century a new Sun style was propagated by Sun Lutang, a master of the earlier internal martial arts.

The taiji form of 128 postures takes about 30 minutes to perform, although there is no set speed. Our approach to the performance of the postures is to go softly, slowly and continuously. So the time to complete the form may shorten to 25 minutes, but it could balloon out to 40 minutes. This long taiji form is divided into seven distinct cycles of movement. There is some repetition in the cycles, for example, the fourth cycle is a repetition of the third cycle, and there are particular postures which are repeated at various points throughout the form.

The traditional way of learning the long form as we call it, is to go out day after day and week after week and simply follow the teacher. If the student forgets a move, then they wait for the next class to focus on that move and then return home to consolidate what they know. This is how a student progresses. However, this way of learning is not so easy to apply in our modern setting. This is why we use the five flowing exercises to introduce taiji to students. These five flowings as well being a complete set in themselves, are the building blocks of the longer taiji form and appear at various points during the long form. We have already noted the correspondence between the five flowings and the physical organs. There are also lists of other correspondences between them, such as the seasons, foods, and emotions etc.

When I learned taiji from Simon, he emphasised the philosophic benefit of taiji. He accepted that it was not for everybody. He used his taiji to enrich his healing art which allowed him to open his door to anybody in need. This form with its 128 postures has such a rich and long relationship with the natural philosophy as expressed in the Yi Jing. That is why he would encourage students to go back to the original sources: to read the *Dao De Jing*, written by Lao Zi; *The Inner Chapters* by Zhuang Zi; and the *Yi Jing*. Of course, we may benefit from reading the work of commentators over the centuries but Simon was a big one for always going back to the original source documents.

Simon drew the distinction between classical and functional taiji and emphasised that our taiji was functional. We were not going to enter taiji competitions and win prizes for perfectly executed forms. We were about getting ourselves moving, about using our taiji to flow our energy for health, and using the moving meditation to relax and energise ourselves.

I had a friend who learned taiji privately in Sydney. He said his teacher never once referred to philosophy. But the teacher was highly adept with the one inch punch where he could bounce a person across a room with a simple nudge. Such stories allowed me to appreciate the form I was learning. Simon had once demonstrated the one inch punch to a group of senior students at his house one Saturday afternoon, but that was the only time I ever saw him demonstrate it in all the years I was with him.

There are so many gems buried in the taiji form that make up part of its logic. For example, I discovered one day that neither hand crosses the centre line of the body. Now this is built into the design of taiji and one day a student will discover this for themselves. But a teacher may instruct the student to not let their hands cross the centre line of the body. But the best teacher may not be so explicit, preferring to encourage the student to focus on the movement of the whole body knowing they will make such discoveries along the way. There are many such treasure in the taiji form.

Simon often came back to the argument that the form was the way to communicate taiji, but the great power of taiji was always in its formless application. We don't want to be limited to using taiji to when we are doing the postures themselves. We want to be able to use our taiji experience any place and any time. For example, we can do our qi breathing and relax ourselves even as we are sitting in an airplane seat. We don't feel limited. We may be in an uncomfortable social situation where it would be highly inappropriate to throw a one inch punch. But we can deal with people in a firm but gentle way. This is what formless taiji is.

A good form is much like a Chinese watercolour painting. There is enough detail there to recognise images, and communicate feelings and yet there is no effort to replicate or represent objects or people or places in their entirety. It can become a beautiful example of the balance of form and formless. This is what Lao Zi describes as the way of no way which we will explore in more detail later.

To explore the philosophy of taiji does not mean that we ignore its physical side, even as a form of self-defence. Our school does have some almost humorous stories of how students have drawn on their taiji as self-defence. For example, one student was assailed by half a dozen young guys in a seedy part of an inner suburb of Sydney. This student was not the fighting type but he began using the movements like 'hand play with the clouds' and he was able to curl away and repel the young guys through this continuous circular motion which may have startled them as much as anything. Of course, people practise self-defence in great detail and it instills amazing confidence and should never be undervalued.

One day before class Simon was giving a talk about the value of not opposing force, but directing it from the centre, essentially the argument for strength in softness. One of his senior female students raised the question: 'But what about if your husband is hitting you? Do you just not fight back?' Simon reaffirmed: 'The most important thing we can do is to go into our centre and flow.' It sounded like a cryptic answer and domestic violence is a highly contentious issue in our country today. However, this student later described to me how the next time the situation arose, she did as she described 'go into her centre', felt totally empty and when her husband hit her, she bounced across the room and hit the wall. She said this event shocked her husband more than anyone and that was the last time he ever touched her. A cycle was broken and she moved out of that situation soon after.

Once a student had learned the long form with Simon, Simon guided them through a centring process. This could be anywhere between 28 and 100 days where the student focussed solely on their centre, the dan tian point, located seven centimetres below the navel and also called the elixir field in Chinese medicine. This process leads the student to look beyond the form, while using it to build their power of focus. After the 28 or how ever many days, the student was guided to direct all that focussed energy out to their extremities, to express all that they had collected. Each generation of Simon's students experienced this differently. For example, one early group were encouraged to take one month to feel their taiji form as heavy as a mountain. This was followed by the next month of where they flowed lightly like a mountain stream.

At Simon's place on weekends we also studied the two supplementary taiji exercises: Pushing Hands and Pushing Body. We began with Pushing Body, a solo exercise consisting of eight distinct moves which are repeated on the left side and the right side. We use this exercise to energise and strengthen our body and it is a great model of how simplicity can contain such complexity. On the Pushing Body exercise, which I still practise regularly, I recall how I saw each of the eight moves as self-defensive, almost imaginary engagements with an attacker. But now, I see them as eight postures, each with a different mood, on how we deal with any situation in our environment. These moods are linked to the eight trigrams and I have written more about this detail elsewhere (*TAO Total Person and One World*).

After the above strengthening and energising exercise, we practised Pushing Hands exercise where we team up with another person and push against them as they, in turn, push against us, as we focus on the harmony of the flow between us. We exercise our firmness and gentleness as we sensitised to the person we are flowing with. This is a key taiji self-defence exercise and essential part of taiji.

It was almost in passing, that Simon showed us what he described as joint and tendon exercises. I recall the names as he taught them, Xisui Jing, Yijin Jing and Daoyin Jing. We build them into our warm up regime, but it was only many years later that I discovered these exercises have their own illustrious history reputed to go back to Boddidharma (also known as Damo) the man who introduced Shaolin to China from India in 527 AD. This was yet another illustration of how inspired was the taiji that Simon shared with his students. It just seemed like it had no end of surprise: it was so complete and yet seemed inexhaustible.

To finish this chapter, try the following activity: Based on the detailed description in the early part of this chapter, do the Hand Play with the Clouds exercise for 3-5 minutes. This exercise will reveal to you how all that wordy description is so different to actually simply doing it. The words help to get you started, but the direct experience is so different. If you are a visual person, search on youtube for this exercise and follow the instructor. The aim of getting you to sample this taiji exercise is to get you to feel your whole body moving as you stand on the same spot, to feel your weight shifting from one foot to the other, and to simply be aware of your centre of gravity as your body moves.

8 Energy or qi

I first learned about the phenomenon of energy within the context of a Western science education. The word, or rather the thing that it signifies, expanded with my exposure to the philosophy underlying taiji. This chapter is a continuation of an account of the experience of non-Chinese person learning a Chinese health art.

Over the past few decades, many highly qualified doctors and physicists have sought to find common ground between theoretical Western physics and Eastern mysticism. Eminent authors such as Fritjof Kapra, Gary Zukav, Deepak Chopra and others have written eloquently and in great depth about the one human reality which lies behind such different perspectives on life and how the history across all cultures has been an expression of this truth. Central to many of those accounts is the way energy is understood. But being arguments presented in books, much of this mind-expanding knowledge often remains academic and its translation into lived human experience cannot be guaranteed.

Most of us learned in middle school the law of conservation of energy which states that energy can neither be created nor destroyed. It sounds dramatic, perhaps epic, and stirs our imagination to think about what fuels the universe in both its big and small sweeps. But it is very much a law for physicists and not one that easily lends itself to helping us much in our daily activities. With such an epic law as this, it is easy to understand why it seems so hard for any investigation into the phenomenon of energy to find a satisfactory starting point. So I intend to dive straight in from where I am, in the true spirit of phenomenology.

My first memory of having energy explained to me was in my physics class in high school, a rather conventional affair. Here I learned that energy is a nonphysical quantity used to perform work or create heat. It is internationally measured in joules, though it can also be measured in ergs, calories, British thermal units, or kilowatt hours. When we say work is a function of energy, we are essentially saying that energy, though nonphysical, has an obvious effect in the physical world. And then we have all these formulae for calculating kinetic and potential energy.

But, in my learning experience, the concept of energy largely remained confined to the field of science. Energy for me remained synonymous with the idea of fuel and of course in the early seventies, the energy crisis was all about the supply of fuel for our cars and other industrial processes. I also recall when I was in high school we could buy glucose powder in cardboard boxes which when made into a drink was promised to give us more energy.

We did have some exposure to more speculative physics, perhaps the most well known equation in physics being Albert Einstein's $E=mc^2$ which proposed that energy is matter and matter is energy. We may ponder on how our views about life would change if we really understood this formula, but our dominant social imperative is to deal with the immediate physical world and so this is also primarily a formula for the advanced physics laboratory. Energy remained in the domain of science just as spirit remained within the domain of religion.

Introducing taiji to new students, Simon explained the concept of qi, or energy, and the part it plays in health and essentially how we can direct it with our mind. I will recreate a demonstration of his further below.

But first, to gain a clearer understanding of the word qi, let's go back to the ideogram within its Chinese character. The simplified character for qi is 气, derived from the traditional character 氣, an image of steam coming off rice. It symbolises the energy radiating from an object. In this image we have the separation of yin and yang, the creation of high and low.

Basic to taiji philosophy is the proposition that we live in two worlds, one is the yang or physical world and the other is the yin or nonphysical. The eternal relationship between the physical and nonphysical worlds is that the physical is ever becoming nonphysical and the nonphysical is ever becoming physical, yin ever becomes yang and yang ever becomes yin, and as part of this process, energy or qi is generated.

Not being brought up in a Chinese culture, we probably don't appreciate how common the word qi is in everyday use, and how it is so freely attributed to the natural world. For example, the Chinese word for weather, tianqi 天气, translates literally as 'the energy of the sky'. But as in all Chinese language, a word needs to be seen in context. So qi can also mean air or gas. When looking at Chinese language, we always need to know the context to understand the full meaning of the word being used.

As explained in an earlier chapter, the flow of this qi in the context of vital energy is essential to health, and a major goal in Chinese medicine is to ensure this qi flows freely through the body. The purpose of taiji is facilitate that flow through all the organs of the body using a series of physical movements.

As mentioned, we began and ended each taiji class with a breathing meditation exercise where we would breathe out to our feet, to our hands and the top of our head. This exercise served to energise and sensitise our body.

Simon would demonstrate the flow of qi by asking students, one at a time, to put out their palm opened and with his hand about 30 centimetres away, he would focus his fingers and slowly wave his hand up and down, directing his qi onto the person's palm which they could feel as warmth. This was one of several demonstrations of taiji which Simon occasionally performed in formal classes.

One regular demonstration of his was the unbendable arm. Each student was asked to put their arm out horizontally at shoulder level and while fully relaxed breathe out to their hands. While the muscles are relaxed another person cannot bend that first person's arm because of the qi energy flowing through it. They were always humorous moments at Sydney Uni when Simon invited several of the largest fellows from the fitness section of the Gym to come in and try and bend his arm. He would be standing relaxed and talking to the group of students as four or five strong men sought to bend his arm but were never able to budge him at all.

We also used a posture 'brushing the swallow's tail' where we imagine a bird sitting on our wrist and we brush its imaginary tail with the other hand. This hand comes close enough to the wrist the feel a band of warmth coming from the arm. Energy as that which produces heat is a sound definition according to the physics text books.

But this is not simple mechanical energy, this is a bioenergy. It is not my purpose in this book to convince others of the existence of bioenergy and the many ways it can enhance our life experience. There are already many wonderful works available which address this issue. And they are a valid part of my taiji learning experience.

One such work is that of Greek author, Kosta Danaos. In the late eighties, I recall watching a documentary on television called *Ring of Fire: An Indonesian Odyssey* where the two presenters visited a qi healer in Java, Indonesia who went by the name of John Chang. I remember this well because I recorded this episode on VHS video tape. John Chang, who used qi, or body electricity, to heal people who came to him, gave a demonstration of the power of his qi. From a distance, he ignited a crumpled sheet of newspaper. I was happy to know that such people existed and thought my video recording would be great to show friends in the future. Kosta Danaos reacted differently. He decided to go and find John Chang and study under him. Trained in engineering but with a personal interest in both European and Eastern esoteric traditions, Kosta took up the challenge of presenting John Chang's skill to the world and elaborating examples of such skill and knowledge within his own tradition, drawing on both the Orthodox religious tradition as well as ancient Greek writings. His two books read as passionate wake up calls to a world in which, he claims, the forgotten side of ourselves has been taken away from us.

I think Kosta would agree that his target reader was the serious seeker of knowledge, one who wanted to reclaim that side of themselves they have been denied by an education which gears most people for slotting into the present economy not the better world that many of us can imagine.

I feel less motivated to convince anybody of anything. I simply want to share my story with others on their journey, and I hope it has something to offer them. Embedded is quite a detailed story of taiji, but running in tandem with this is the story of a seeker feeling his way forward in the late twentieth and early twenty-first century.

I marvel how energy has assumed a god-like mystery status. It can be so many things to so many people. The thing is that energy can radiate across such a range of frequencies and wherever it lies on this range it is still called energy. I am of a generation who will not flinch when he listens to people in conversation talk about cosmic energy, psychic energy, sexual energy and so on.

In European philosophy, there are threads of a tradition of bio-energy, For example in the early years of the twentieth century French philosopher, Henri Bergson (1859-1941), proposed a philosophy of vitalism based on a vital energy force which underlies physical matter (elan vital). This can be traced to the German philosopher, Gottfried Leibniz, who also proposed a type of bio-energy. But Bergson's idea was met with resistance by contemporary mainstream thinkers. However, current concepts of organicism in the field of biology and life sciences owe a lot to Bergson's contribution to the subject.

Another great pioneer in the field of bioenergy was US Professor of Anatomy, Harold Saxton Burr (1889-1973). In the early 1930s, he proposed an electro-dynamic theory of life. After successfully measuring the output of electric current in corn, he proposed that 'electricity seems to bridge the gap between the lifeless world and living matter...electricity is one of the fundamental factors in all living systems, just as it is in the non-living world.' He went on to develop the concept of fields of life (L-fields) which was cooly received by the establishment, considered by some to be ahead of its time.

Numerous individuals have devoted their lives to investigation into the phenomenon of energy beyond what is taught in formal settings. While the research findings of such individuals can be enriching, any knowledge gained is not easily integrated into the mainstream body of learning, because it appears to conflict with core beliefs held by science today, particularly in the lines it draws between mind and matter.

Many of the sixties generation are familiar with the name of the famous Brazilian 'surgeon of the rusty knife', José Pedro de Freita, also known as Zé Arigó, who is said to have treated more than two million people between 1956 and 1971. In 1968, a scientific investigation team of six doctors and eight other scientists headed by New York neurologist, Andrija Puharich, investigated his work and provided first hand accounts of operations conducted by him. Despite carrying out thousands of major operations with rusty scissors, he had a record of no infections and no post-operative complications. It is fair to say that he was working on a nonphysical level that regular science struggled to explain.

Another interesting example of the blurring of lines between mind and matter is the research by Japanese scientist, Masaru Emoto, who has demonstrated that water has the capacity for memory. His work focused on the study of crystal patterns formed by particular samples of water once they were frozen. He has demonstrated in repeat experiments that water shows evidence of receiving and holding the mental vibrations projected by human beings. Emoto claims his greater mission is to show people that we have a more intimate relationship with our environment than we have been traditionally taught.

On the subject of memory, we may remember that energy is simply coded information. This is a reason why energy is important for the physical body, it contains enormous amounts of memory data. Some speculate that we have a point in our body where we have the history of all human experience. This is sometimes referred to as the akashic record, another word for our centrepoint.

Many people have pursued bio-energy research at great cost to themselves. The Austrian-born psychiatrist, Willhelm Reich, a student of Sigmund Freud, migrated to the United States where he developed a whole system based on sexual energy which he termed orgone energy. Apart from the work he conducted with individuals, including technology to accumulate orgone energy from the environment, he proposed revolutionary views on how the energy of the sexual sphere interacted with broader society. He claimed that dictatorships and authoritarian governments sought to harness the sexual energy of the masses and divert that energy for other projects, eg Hitler's goal of domination through war. Of course, we are familiar with the tradition of the Catholic Church which sought to control the sexuality of its most trusted members. The US authorities suspected Reich, a fervent advocate of freedom, was perpetrating fraud with his orgone accumulators, and he was imprisoned where he eventually died. Controversially, six tons of his publications were burned by order of the court at that time.

So we can see from the sketch in this chapter that this phenomenon we call energy intersects with so many different levels of life, from science to religion to sexuality to politics to mind. It is both new and old. But the human being has shown again and again it will keep asking questions and will keep reaching out for new understandings and will accept no limitation. With this knowledge, we can see that the suggestion that we use mind more and force less is a steady but reliable way forward into the unknown.

Knowledge about energy alone will never be enough. If ignorance is an energy which seeks to conserve itself as per our high school learning about the nature of energy, then our goal surely must be to both understand energy and know how to direct it.

In earlier chapters, I expressed a concern that scientists had, in a sense, hypnotised us with their dogma, their small bag of truths about the world. I see now, that my disappointment was not with science itself. It was with the fact that there was a lot more to know and discover. Science portrays itself as complete when there is so much more to know. As a simple example, consider the function of the eye. We are taught that the eye is a sense organ which receives stimulation from external sources ie that it is a receptive organ. But there is also a long held esoteric science that proposes the eye gives off an energy, that when we look at objects whether near or far, that we are transversing distance at the energy level to have some sort of contact with that object. Leonardo a Vinci was a strong advocate of the transmission of soul energy via vision. Of course, our clarity of vision depends on the amount of light available, so both the conditions of transmission and reception are involved. I look forward to the day when science becomes more complete.

9 Zhang San Feng

In one of my earliest taiji classes, I learned that taiji was developed in China about seven hundred years ago by a nobleman named Zhang San Feng, Zhang of the Three Mountain Peaks. It was a simple enough story.

With our focus on learning the basics of taiji movement and breathing, our teacher only had the time to tell us this version of Zhang's story: That he was well-versed in the three doctrines of China (Daoism, Confucianism and Buddhism) and was also trained in Shaolin boxing, the most esteemed martial art of the day (the Shaolin Temple on Song Mountain had been the hub of Shaolin gong fu for over a thousand years); that Zhang wasn't satisfied with the skills and knowledge he had gained up till that point in life and so he dropped everything and went to live as a hermit in the Wu Dang Mountains; and that thirteen years later he returned with the taiji form with its emphasis on mind and the development of strength through softness.

As a student new to taiji, I accepted this story on its face value. After all, I was only attending an introductory course and this amount of information served its purposes for me. I was satisfied that taiji was developed by a person who had searched and studied hard for a better way of being, a person who had developed a calisthenic exercise which also doubled up as a meditation as well as potentially being the deadliest martial art on earth if one had the patience to learn. And it seemed good that this happened long ago so that the art had the time to be distilled and refined and tested over centuries.

On another evening, before class started, my teacher told us an anecdote about how Zhang created the taiji form while living as a hermit. One day, while meditating in his house, he heard an unusual noise coming from the courtyard. From his window, he saw a snake hissing at a crane that had flown down to attack it. The snake turned away from the crane's sword-like beak and beat at the crane's neck with its tail. The crane defended its neck with its right wing and then the snake twined itself around the crane's legs. The crane lifted its left leg and lowered its left wing to help it attack the snake, but although it stabbed again and again with its beak it could never catch the snake, which always twisted out of reach. In the end they both gave up from sheer tiredness and the crane went back to its branch while the snake crawled into a hole in the same tree. This scene gave Zhang the idea of the interplay of yin and yang as it applied to physical movement: that the strong becomes the yielding and the yielding becomes the strong. It was this event that inspired him to come up with the form of taiji.

As new students learning the form, we could relate to this because as we moved our weight from one foot to the other, back and forth, we were being trained to feel the interplay of tension and relaxation, left foot, right foot, left foot, right foot, a model of yin and yang rhythmically giving way to each other, a model of how strength is born out of softness.

A few years later, while doing honours research at Sydney University, I discovered that the story of Zhang San Feng was far more complicated than that account given in my introductory taiji course. Although historical records refer to Zhang as a Daoist Immortal of the Ming Dynasty (1368-1644), he wasn't generally recognised as the founder of taiji until the early 1900s. This snippet of information stimulated me to dig further to know how his present status as a taiji hero might have come about. Especially as, in modern day China, Zhang has become an all time kung fu hero due largely to contemporary novels and films about his life and deeds.

To read early accounts of Zhang San Feng and his life is to become enchanted with a person larger than life can imagine. He is said to have been a tall man who looked like he had the longevity of a turtle and the immortality of a crane. He had enormous eyes and ears, a beard which seemed to bristle with blade-like strands, and hair tied in a knot at the back of his head. He is also said to have always worn a single cassock, and a bamboo hat, and he could sleep in the snow without catching a cold. He could also eat huge quantities of food at one sitting or fast for months at a time. Stories also mention how he could climb mountains as if flying.

Beware that there are critics who claim any acceptance of Zhang as the founder of taiji is based on a myth and that no good student of taiji should engage in such foolhardy ignorance. They lament how the younger generation of martial arts students are so content to live in unquestioning blissful ignorance. Stanley Henning is one such critic. He postulates that the Zhang San Feng myth surfaced around 1910 as an immediate response to the surge in popularity of Shaolin martial arts that went back to Bodhidarma. The alternative martial art, which originated from Wu Dang Mountain, was losing ground and had to come up with a better story about its origins. But these critics sound very much like people who would like to put a man in a Santa Claus suit in prison for not being the true Santa.

This is where I don my phenomenologist's hat. I intend to suspend judgement and stay neutral as I examine the phenomenon of Zhang San Feng. I must give this amazing historical phenomenon a chance to make its case. While I acknowledge there is an important question of historical or literal truth at stake, I would like to keep my mind open to other perspectives about the story that may be beneficial to us. I want to be open to other possible metaphorical and perhaps metaphysical truths that may lie within the story as well.

In researching this chapter I acknowledge the research work of German sinologist, Anna Seidel, a recognised world expert on the history of Daoism. In 1970, she published a paper, *A Taoist Immortal of the Mind Dynasty: Chang San-Feng*. A more scholarly analysis reveals that our Zhang of the Three Mountain Peaks became the founder of taiji in three discrete steps. The earliest records of Zhang San Feng speak of him as a Taoist master. There was no reference to fighting arts, let alone taiji. Zhang was generous enough to give himself the title of Master of Triple Abundance Capable of Endurance and Preserving Harmony. In 1459 the Emperor bestowed him with another title: The Immortal Penetrating Mystery and Revealing Transformation. Even the story behind this title becomes cloudy as some say the Emperor was seeking to lure Zhang to the capital to help him govern the empire, while others say it was a ruse to track down the heir of a previous dynasty who was reputed to be alive in the area where Zhang lived.

In the 1500s Wang Zong Yue, a taiji master, claimed to have a treatise written by Zhang San Feng which had been handed down to him by his teachers. Wang imputed Zhang San Feng as being the founder of the inner school of martial arts. With the deft use of a smart mind, the fighter knew how to locate the opponent's weak spots and immobilise them so they didn't need to rely on greater strength. The internal art, which defied the expectation that the stronger opponent would defeat the weaker opponent, was more than the achievement of an eccentric individual. It was a body of teaching that could be shared within schools. And its founder was declared to be Zhang San Feng.

For many generations, taiji survived as a family secret. It was kept within the walls of the Chen family village in Henan Province. In the 1800s, for various reasons, taiji spread outside that village and attracted wider interest from other parts of China. Not a lot of information about taiji could be found outside that Chen family and to extract information from them required both a great deal of loyalty and a big investment of time.

Zhang's elevated status was further enhanced by a Taoist spirit writing cult in the nineteenth century who claimed to communicate with him through planchette writing, the equivalent to the Western ouija board. Members of this cult published the complete works of Zhang San Feng based on recordings of their séance communications with him.

As mentioned above, in the early 1900s the time was ripe for this eccentric to become bestowed with the honour of having introduced taiji to the world. Prior to the 1960s, taiji was rarely taught outside the Chinese community. Once it was unleashed onto the Western world, Zhang San Feng's role as the founder of taiji gained the status of fact.

After doing taiji daily over many years, I'm okay with the Zhang San Feng story. I view it as a cultural agglomerate. In geology, an agglomerate is a coarse accumulation of large blocks of volcanic material. It contains a high proportion of individually-shaped rocks which may or may not have fused together under heat.

We in the Western world place a premium on truth, but we don't pause to consider that it may be only one ingredient in the mix of a good story. Truth is sometimes reached with a leap of the imagination.

Seidel's careful combing of historical references reveals numerous claims about Zhang San Feng linking him to the art of longevity; the love of nature and abhorrence of social conventions; the art of war; the path to wealth and prosperity; health; the patron saint of comedy and eccentric; the art of magic; the skill of long distance walking.

Zhang is a remarkable story with lots of delicious detail. I could even liken it to the long form of taiji itself, which is like a bellows producing more and more over time. The story is about a man who had a lot and wanted more, a man who created something beautiful but yet never forced it on anyone. A story of a man who had broken the bonds of society and wandered freely to enjoy life in the way he saw fit. He did not oppose others, or even criticise them.

It may be prose, it may be poetry, it may be nonfiction, it may be fiction, but the story of Zhang San Feng is part of the taiji legacy, and while we should not feel compelled to embrace the stories about his life, it is no reason not to explore taiji and its heritage for its great value in our celebration of health and wellbeing.

10 My teacher

There is a saying that describes how a taiji master appears to those around them: 'When I am close I am very close and when I am far I am very far.' This is an apt description of how Simon, my teacher, impacted the lives of myself and many of my fellow students. In so many cases, he allowed people to come very close to him, where he could exercise a powerful influence on their life path, but he was always soon on his way to his next appointment. Of course he may be far from us now, but the memory of him, the energy that he radiated during these exchanges, remains very close.

In the late eighties, I recall working in a health food store in Bondi Junction on one quiet morning when I got talking with a customer. I told this customer, whom I had never met before, how I enjoyed doing taiji each morning before work. He was curious and asked me who my teacher was. I mentioned Simon's name. His face lit up and he said: 'Wow, that guy! He saved my marriage.' There were so many stories floating around about Simon's sublime impact on people's lives.

Before the start of our Sydney Uni taiji classes, we would wait near the entrance to the auditorium as the previous exercise class emptied. During this time, Simon liked to chit-chat, as he described it, with early-comers, sharing his enthusiasm for taiji. In one of the early weeks of the first session, I was next to him and asked him whether he reckoned taiji would help me give up smoking.

He paused before he began. 'It will help. But not by fighting it, taiji will make your body stronger and smoking will fall away by itself.' In this first conversation with him, he had shared the essence of taiji: find success through non-fighting and non-resistance.

After that he laughed. 'Believe me, I know, when I worked at the brewery, I used to smoke and drink, and my liver must have been this big.' His right hand gestured out from the side of his body as if his liver reached out the length of his arm. I discovered Simon previously worked as an organic chemist at Tooth's Brewery closer to the city up on Broadway.

Even as I took it all in, satisfied with the answer, I had the feeling he could see through me, knew I was asking the question perhaps to be sociable, maybe to overcome nervousness in his presence, and that he knew I had taken up taiji for more reasons than just giving up smoking. We both knew I was there for a much bigger dream. Part of Simon's teaching was to weave the long term into the short term and the short term into the long term, and this was typical Simon in action. It was almost coded language, but just as when we did taiji postures one arm forms part of a large circle, is more linear, and the other arm is part of a small circle, is more curved, Simon could talk about the big circle and the small circle and we all knew what he was talking about. We knew our taiji would help us into the centre of the big circle.

Incidentally, I gave up smoking some time later, effortlessly. I was sick one night, had a fever, and gastro upset, and the next morning I felt fantastic. I wasn't interested in smoking again. And I never feared people who smoked around me. If anybody nearby smoked, I reckoned it was their business not mine. And if anyone asked me about smoking, I would tell them to enjoy it while they can because one day when they no longer smoked, it would be nothing but a memory.

In that first year of classes at the University of Sydney, two medicine students from Hong Kong, Francis and Louis, were members of our class. The way they sparred with one another before and sometimes during class, it was obvious they already had much exposure to martial arts. I recall Louis one night explaining to me about the role of a teacher in the martial arts world. He said that, while studying with a teacher, students often love their teacher more than their own father. This is because of the powerful influence they have in guiding their students into what is essentially a whole new world of being. In a very unassuming way, Simon generated enormous trust and confidence amongst his students as well as his patients who I will write more about later, and due to the way he was so dedicated to his art, I found this true for myself and many of Simon's senior students.

Simon migrated to Australia from Indonesia in the early sixties. He was born into a Chinese family in Jakarta in 1939. Before he was a teenager, Simon and his family had witnessed: the Japanese occupation of

Indonesia; the end of Dutch colonial rule with the bloody fighting that accompanied it; the rise of a new Indonesian nationalism; the threat of Communism which at that time was feared would knock down country after country as part of the dreaded 'domino effect'; and also the general climate of suspicion of Chinese in Indonesia for both ethnic and political reasons. With such turbulence in his formative years, I can understand him being drawn to a vision of dynamic meditation and the accompanying Daoist concepts of quietness in movement and movement in quietness. He was far from the tradition of a small taiji village. By the early sixties, Simon's father decided to send him to study in Australia and perhaps start a new life there.

Simon's father was a Hakka Chinese. Hakka are the guest people, people from other places, who were often given the most un-arable land when they migrated to a new region. This experience helped shape them to become a hardworking yet cheerful and very proud people. There are many Chinese people of Hakka ancestry who have occupied high places in recent history. For example, Lee Kuan Yew, the founder of modern Singapore was Hakka, and Sun Yat Sen, the founder of the People's Republic of China, was also Hakka.

In his teenage years, before he moved overseas, Simon involved himself in the normal activities of schoolwork and sport and physical activity. He was a competition swimmer and he studied Shaolin martial arts. He once told us that he did a correspondence course on qi gong meditation and that he used his qi gong to prepare himself before his swimming races. He said he overdid it before one race meeting and fainted. His father warned him off his meditation activity for the time being. However, that course certainly had a formative influence on his future taiji interests.

Simon completed his matriculation studies three times: in a Chinese school, in an Indonesian school and then in an Australian school. He graduated from Sydney University in 1966 with a Bachelor of Science degree. He later did other postgraduate studies in microbiology and biochemistry.

In the early seventies, he went back to Indonesia with his family to pursue some business opportunities. It was while he was there that he attended bagua and taiji classes. During the course of learning taiji in Indonesia, he was practicing in a park one evening when he was hit by a runaway truck. He ended up in hospital for months because of the damage to his legs. This included his nerves being severed near the knee, and he says it was his taiji teacher's guidance that helped him recover so completely from that injury, including helping his nerves regrow. Simon's taiji teacher also practised Chinese medicine from his home. He introduced Simon to the art during the course of his taiji study with him.

In much the same way that I felt my life was preparing me for my eventual encounter with taiji, I can now see that Simon too had been through a lot of preparation long before his teacher ever arrived on the scene.

When he came back to Australia, Simon worked as an industrial chemist. At the same time he began to run taiji classes and a small natural health clinic from his home. Taiji, martial arts and oriental philosophy had become trendy in the seventies. Offering a very refined version of the art of taiji, Simon quickly began to attract a stream of sensitive people. Living in Campsie, where he kept his family of wife and three children, he used a spare room by the front door of his house as the clinic room while he also taught some taiji exercises and spoke to students and visitors out in a leafy backyard.

In the late seventies/early eighties, he sought to expand his activities. He began to teach at several universities and other institutions around Sydney. For a few years, he taught taiji to future actors at NIDA (National Institute of Dramatic Arts) located on the UNSW campus. As he built his school, Simon went out to introduce taiji to many new groups and then in his own locality he ran his advanced class: in-depth taiji meditation where Simon sought to train teachers. So he had the dual operation of taking senior students out to learn to teach in the various city locations and also bringing students back to the Canterbury classes when they were ready.

Simon, while incredibly focussed on his sharing the taiji idea, was amazingly flexible and a great communicator. Even in the same class, Simon could be guiding his senior students in the long taiji form, providing counsel as to health, physical and mental, as well metaphysical to each and all in a very personal way. On the same evening, as students took turns to lead the group, he may sit with one of the student's children, perhaps five years old, who was drawing and colouring in as they waited for their parent to finish class, and Simon could hold a rich and engaging conversation with the child before switching back to the in-depth meditation class. Simon often spoke about the value of being attached and detached at the same time.

He began his weekend clinic from his house in Campsie. He never advertised that clinic. It grew by word of mouth. His taiji classes became a main source for his patients as students would bring their family and friends for help. When the clinic became too crowded, Simon borrowed the premises of a naturopathic clinic from his friend in Kingsgrove on Saturdays. This clinic had three rooms, and Simon had all three rooms fully occupied with patients as he moved from one to the other, like a chess master playing multiple games of chess at the same time.

From the early eighties, Simon managed a health food store located on campus at the University of New South Wales. The store was called The Nut House. At that time, health foods stores were outlets for bulk grains and dried fruits and nuts etc. It was a good business when we consider the number of student share houses. Health food was an important plank in Simon's natural health proposition. So he was building a small empire, based on his exercise classes, his natural health clinic and his health food store.

In 1984, Simon and eight of his senior students embarked on a venture to open another health food store in Rozelle. The venture had several goals. Firstly, it was an opportunity to increase Simon's buying power for his shop at the university; also it gave members of our group greater exposure to the health food industry; it was also part of our effort to build a school of health and healing. It was called The Rozelle Health Food Centre. It had a large spare room inside the shop and that would enable the group to expand availability of the clinic to the public. This shop was also a short walk from a dis-used church which operated as a community centre where we taught taiji on Friday nights and ran workshops some weekends. The shop lasted for several years before the lease expired and was not renewed as members pursued other projects.

Those times were a playful combination of the need to address the immediate business practicalities of running a health food store and also building our school, of teaching taiji and developing the clinic. Most of the time these activities were separated. But part of the fun was to switch from one mode to the other. We were all for learning to harmonise the yin and yang sides of life.

I recall late one Saturday afternoon in the shop. The long day of firstly opening the shop at 8.30am and then helping with the clinic in the afternoon was followed by a business meeting. As we were wrapping up, Simon walked over to a member of our team, exactly in front of where I was seated. He raised his right hand and patted this team member of the shoulder. What I saw was a ball of white energy come from Simon's hand, entering the shoulder, the ball flew straight into my team member's abdomen, that point called the dan tian. I had seen this ball of energy as clearly as anything I have ever seen, but I had nothing to compare it to, never having ever seen anything like it before. I felt as though Simon was personally demonstrating this skill right there in front of me. That one moment of observation captured perfectly how the transfer of energy is done, worth more than hours of trying and studying qi gong, and yet perhaps I would never had seen it if I had not spent years studying this either. I never mentioned this to anyone, and as I write, this is the first time I have shared it with another. There were a series of these moments during my time with Simon, rare, but when they happened, they just tore away the veil of what we are used to seeing and experiencing in our normal world.

Simon and several of his senior students made several attempts to build a platform to present to the world. Tai Chi Acupressure Organisation (TAO) and later Natural Health Technology and Research (NHTR) None of these jelled before Simon decided in 1988 to go overseas and establish his natural healing clinic in Jakarta. Again, he was off to his next appointment. This was an intense time in his life. At that clinic, he had an open door policy, where he would admit patients any time of day or night. He came back to Australia, in 1994, feeling very exhausted.

From Simon's high times, he withdrew into retirement very slowly. His first step was to leave Sydney and move down to the Illawarra. Here he still taught some relaxation and some martial arts classes to locals as well operating a limited clinic, again in the front room of his house. He continued to be busy in the local area with his membership of the Illawarra Lapidary Club and also his attendance of line dancing classes at the local Leagues Club.

After suffering a fall, Simon lightened his activities, spending more time at home, still always happy to see visitors, whether they be new or old faces. After suffering several strokes, he became confined to his bed and was so fortunate to be in the care of his wife.

In January 2018 I received a call that Simon had passed away. While he may have seemed far away from the physical point of view, I recalled many wonderful moments in my relationship with him. I remembered the intensely busy time when we were setting up the shop in Rozelle. The day before opening, I recall receiving a call from him at home early in the morning, reminding me to bring something or other, his voice so brisk and full of energy. That morning was spent in the shop with Simon, the director of operations. Come afternoon, we opened the clinic doors, another demanding time serving those in need. After that, we went to a restaurant and Simon was still so inexhaustible with his words and ideas. After being a student of Simon's for but a short time before, I pondered on how amazing it was to be in the company of such a great teacher like this all in the course of a single day. When he was close he was very close!

11 The clinic

When I spoke at Simon's funeral service, one of the anecdotes I shared was of a lady who visited his naturopathy clinic in Campsie in 1981. I had not long started attending this clinic.

Her name was Grace, a white-haired lady, in her late sixties, a little overweight, a kindly Aussie grandmother whose face was branded with experience, its broad horizontal lines suggesting a person who could appreciate the life of today when compared with those difficult days gone by, but still a woman with a keen eye, as if she was the matriarch who knew the personalities and idiosyncrasies of each and every member of her extended family as well as how to deal with them most effectively, for she was as straight a talker as you would ever meet. To be bent over with arthritis, as she was, was not her natural state and this was causing her a lot of pain.

When she came to the clinic, she couldn't walk from the car to the house but had to be carried by her two sons. After making the obligatory welcoming fuss at the front door, Simon led her into his room with a smile and a hand guiding her to the chair.

She sized Simon up and began. 'I think I'm done for. This pain is killing me.' She had taken all the medicines as prescribed by her doctor, yet still suffered the aches and pains, and was told she would need to learn how to manage the condition as there was little alternative. She continued expressing her dissatisfaction with the advice she had been given by her doctors as Simon checked the pulses on each of her wrists, nodding his head, a gesture of assurance he was listening. He seemed to be listening to both her words and the cries for help coming from the organs of her body which Chinese medicine postulates are expressed in those pulses he was tracking with his fingertips.

Simon eventually took his hands off her wrists and stood in front of her. 'Grace, today we will help ease some of the pain, but we need to clean you up inside, so if you can come and see me two more times four weeks apart, we will have you dancing again. I promise.'

Grace turned to her sons: 'God, wouldn't it be nice if what he says is true.'

Simon put his hand on her shoulder. 'Grace, we have a lot of experience in dealing with arthritis. I stand by my word.'

She couldn't help but smile as she heard those words, be they true or not true. 'If I ever dance again, it'll be a bloody miracle. That's for sure!'

In Chinese medicine, the joints have a strong correspondence with the liver function in the body, and so from the outside Simon would massage points on the liver meridian and from the inside he would recommend some herbal treatment to cleanse and nourish her liver. This was after a general acupressure energy treatment which would lift and refresh her whole body.

Chinese medicine uses the same terms for an organ as Western medicine, but it is more correctly a function, and that function is not fixed to one location but is distributed across every cell in the body, just as the lungs as an organ breathes oxygen, the lung function is extended to every cell. It is the same for the liver, the blood cleansing and building function occurs throughout the whole body.

I was fortunate enough to be there when Grace made her third visit. She was smiling, chirpy and cheerful almost as if Simon had been granted honorary membership to her extended family. I don't know if she got to dance again but after that third visit she walked to her car unassisted, with good posture and a broad smile on her face.

Simon was always telling his students to keep records of such case studies, but what he was practising was a subtle art, an art with so many moving parts, from the sandy paradigm of Chinese medicine to the deft psychology of dealing with each person as they presented, to the mysterious art of reading twelve different pulses on the wrists, to the chemistry and biochemistry of herbs and vitamins he would carefully select and recommend in specific doses, and to the sensitivity required in massage and natural physiotherapy. We all have our first hand experience but very little was kept in the way of systematic records. To us students, Simon would remind us that in the old times the student would carry the bag for the traditional Chinese doctor as he consulted

74

with his patients. Slowly, they would absorb the whole art, putting all those pieces together: monkey see and monkey do.

I mentioned Grace at the service as an example of hundreds of cases I witnessed at that weekend clinic over a period of years. A typical case for Simon was one where the person had given up on their doctor or specialist. They had found little relief, let alone a cure. And so they had been urged by a family member or a friend to at least give Simon a try.

I was endlessly surprised at the number of people in that area who had operations for back problems and yet still suffered back pain. Each time Simon would advise those sufferers that he needed to get the energy flowing through the body before making any physical adjustments. More than once, he used the example of the alignment of iron filings on a sheet of paper with the magnet underneath. It was the energy alignments which was most essential. Many times he suggested we could set up a clinic just to deal with back problems alone and we would have at least an 80 per cent success rate.

Another thing that amazed me was the way his patients would tell stories of how they had spent thousands of dollars on surgery and other treatment all to little benefit and then after a visit to his clinic they would flick a small payment Simon's way as his policy was fee by donation. Some students chided him for this policy but he would explain he wanted to make his clinic available to everybody.

Simon's health clinic and his therapeutic practices have an important part in this book, not only because acupressure therapy is based on the principle of energy flow, the same principle which applies to taiji exercise, but also because it is a clear example of how to apply the idea of 'use mind and not force', ie how we can achieve better health results when we can better read and understand the wisdom of our body so we don't need to use so much force, nay violence, in the course of dealing with sickness. Too often, in forcing a result, we are left to deal with costly and unwanted side effects. When Napoleon Bonaparte said to a group of doctors,'You medical people will have more lives to answer for in the other world than even we generals,' it suggests that the mindless use of force is pervasive across many areas of our society.

In the martial arts context, acupressure therapy offers another lure, for the healing points located on the body, those which allow the energy to flow through it so our organs can breathe and function normally, can also in some cases become killing points when they are struck by an adversary. Even if a student does not wish to injure another, many a martial artist is attracted to the idea of being able to heal themselves if ever their points were ever to become blocked.

I attended Simon's weekend clinic for over six years. He was sharing valuable knowledge about health and taiji and its applications even if we were never to go on and became naturopaths ourselves.

When a person arrived at the clinic, they would be asked to lie down on their stomach on a massage table. Their hands would rest on the table near their head so that we could feel the pulses in the wrists. We would also use an infrared lamp above the sacrum area to warm the body. Firstly, we would do a light muscle massage, usually with an electric massage machine, to help the person relax better so that the pulse readings could be clearer. We then use our fingertips to massage a series of 36 points located along 14 acupressure meridians running along the body. You can visibly see a patient relax and breathe more freely when any such congested points are massaged.

Depending on the condition with the patient and also the outcome of the pulse reading, more attention may be given to one particular part of the body. Once the acupressure massage was over, we did some natural physiotherapy adjustments to the legs. These adjustments work on the hips and the back and are sometimes a coaching exercise for the patient to move more freely. After that, the patient sits up and we would suggest some herbs or vitamins or dietary adjustment. The whole process would take an hour.

Simon didn't oppose modern medicine in itself. There is a lot of benefit to be gained from the innovations and inventions from medical research. His concern was that the people involved in the mainstream medical establishment had a lot to gain by keeping people dependent and effectively sick. The statistic at that time was that over half of the population was on long term pharmaceutical medication. A more recent 2108 report states that nine million Australians take prescription medicines daily. Consultation, treatment and medication are a multi-billion dollar business. But it seems as though it is built on the premise that we can blast our way to health, which just doesn't seem to be working.

In her book, *The Death of a Doctor*, author Sue Williams gives a mind-boggling account of the trial of medically trained doctor, Dr John Harrison, a man who turned to natural methods of healing involving bodywork and psychotherapy rather than operating as a conventional General Practitioner. Harrison built his profile on the promotion of his best-selling book *Love Your Disease, It's Making You Healthy* for which a number of conservatives in the medical establishment showed little appreciation. I often listened to Dr Harrison on regular evening radio segments where he impressed as a highly experienced person devoted to natural health and healing.

Williams, in her book, noted that, at that time, the average GP was prescribing $300,000 worth of medications each year whereas Dr Harrison had only prescribed $79 worth. His case handled by the Health Care Complaints Commission revolved around claims of sexual assault stemming from the touching element of his bodywork modalities. He was barred from practising medicine for life.

While Harrison was in some ways an enlightened doctor, he was also engaged in a strategy of resistance against the status quo. A reminder that, just as if we are chopping wood, it pays to go with the grain. To go against the grain can damage our hands. This is an art we are all learning: the value of paying attention to the energy flow and finding the path of least resistance.

Simon went further to say that doctors superstitiously believed that forcefully making things look right to the naked eye, without accounting for the not so obvious energy disruptions in the body. Simon operated with a naturopathic undertaking of no drugs and no surgery. He was also concerned that across the world, the laws of economics meant that modern medicine, though it may get quick results, would never be available to serve everybody. His offer to the world was a treatment which was cheap and natural. This may of course change at different times.

Any debate about the value of traditional Chinese medicine must factor in belief. If people are in an allowing state of mind, it is more likely to work. And if a person is resistant, there is a lower chance of success. Science will eventually bear this out. We need to accept that people have different belief sets. I recall when I hurt my knee while on a run through a national park. I was running downhill and slid on loose gravel and fell heavily, banged my knee on the ground. It was a physical injury which lingered for some months. One day when I was at the swimming pool, a fellow swimmer was adamant that I should investigate a knee replacement operation because these things happen. But I visited an acupuncture sports therapist who did two sessions of acupuncture within a week and then said there was no need for me to come back. After another week, my knee was as good as it had ever been. I know which option I was happier to take.

Simon once described a case that happened when he was working in Indonesia. An old village head came to him with what he described as a serious problem. He told Simon that everybody in the village had contracted hepatitis but they had no money to buy medicine or get treatment. Simon recommended to him that everybody in the village should drink about 200ml of their own urine first thing every morning. This is probably the ultimate in cheap and tailor-made medicine. Simon later heard from the village head that the hepatitis had quickly been eliminated.

On the subject of urine therapy, some call it the water of life, there is currently a lot of research being done in many universities around the world into its medicinal effects. It has long been used in England by naturopaths who even cite references in the bible to support their case: 'Drink waters out of thine own cistern, and running waters out of thine own well (Proverbs 5:15)'. I have written elsewhere about this subject (RU4UT?). The reason I include the subject here is to demonstrate it as an example of methods to achieve natural health which are effective but which do not fit with the dominant social health paradigm, often a market driven package of beliefs, often determined by those with vested interests. Simon was not concocting methods and techniques, he was using his extensive experience to gather the best of new and old resources available to help patients.

We can only appreciate the amazing advances in technology in recent times and how it has led to better levels of health across the world. But naturopathic medicine will always remind us to see the body as a whole before we break it down into parts. If we don't know how the whole body operates, the energy, the vitality, that binds together all of the various parts, then we can really become tangled in our specialisations. We can have all these wonderful tools and machines and not know how to apply them. In taiji, we learn how we integrate mind, body and breath for health, and Chinese medicine is an extension of this.

In Michael Minick's book about kung fu exercise, he explained in an early chapter that the traditional Chinese doctor was trained to listen to both the patient and their body. Pulse reading was part of this process. But he also noted that there are six important questions which can reliably indicate the health of a person:

1. Are you free from fatigue?
2. Do you sleep soundly?
3. Is your appetite good?
4. Are you good-humoured?
5. Is you memory good?
6. Are you precise in thought and action?

It is easy to be lost in an ocean of indicators and measurements and test results which are all helpful pieces of information but may not add up to much if we can't integrate them. Also, often those pieces of information are not looking at the health resources of the body but actually focus on a weakness or an illness. It pays to maintain our focus on health and ask how we can harness the health and vitality at hand. We will return to the basis of this idea later in the book when we talk about metaphysics and the nature of the world and the human being. In summary, we are perceptive beings and we attract towards us more of what we are giving our attention to, so that the more we focus on health and what's working well in our bodies, the more health we will see, whereas the more we look at illness, the more we will find. So we always have a choice to make.

Returning to Grace's arthritis condition, I do remember words Simon once used in the clinic, that the body, in depositing the acids and waste in the joints was an 'act of love' on the body's part to ensure that they are pushed as far away from the main organs of the body as possible. If we don't understand the body logic, or actually resist it, then we can often worsen the situation. The body has a far greater capacity to rearrange itself than we give it credit for, if only we can learn from it.

12 Sydney Uni

I was in no hurry to complete my Bachelor of Arts degree at Sydney University. All up, I enrolled in philosophy, psychology and anthropology, plus I claimed some credits for a few mathematics subjects from my earlier degree. I chose philosophy and psychology as my co-majors, with the hope of doing an extra honours year in philosophy if my marks were satisfactory.

It can get very circular, the way we wonder why we wonder why, but for a long time after I graduated, I did ponder on what it was that drove me to enrol in a philosophy course at university. Of course, there are many contributing factors: I sometimes think it was my way of shaking off a Catholic education, of replacing years of faith-based indoctrination with some fresher thinking; it could have been that the impressionable young me was living out my uncle's dream, having adopted his hunger to know what in the hell it was all about, and wanting answers to everything from the nature of politics to power to death and meaning; connected to this, it could have been my seizing the opportunity to learn more about my own intellectual, cultural and historical heritage as a foundation for whatever career I would later choose; or maybe, after walking away from a half-finished science degree, I just wanted to take a step back and go more general with my studies until I felt a new direction calling me; more mundanely, it could have been a fun way to pass the time after deciding to go and live under the bright lights of Sydney; then again, it could have been, without my clear knowing at that stage, that I had a rendez-vous with my taiji teacher who started teaching classes at the university the same year that I arrived there.

Whatever the answer, it all worked out well, for the taiji classes I took at the Gym gave me a broader, more life-affirming perspective on my formal philosophy studies, while my philosophy studies enhanced my capacity to absorb and appreciate the taiji idea, as if to nail it down against the backdrop of the western intellectual tradition, to make my taiji learning richer, more robust, more me.

The history of academic philosophy in Australia is a world few have explored. We have long been home to the purveyors of the perennial philosophy, once called Platonists and later idealists; we also have a strong representation from the empiricists who believe in the infallibility of the senses and many of whom dismiss the unknown as unmeasurable and therefore non-existent; there are the logicians who, to me, see life as little more than a battle of wits- all the way to the end; we have the religious folk who strive to theologise their daily life experience; and those whose political position can be traced to either the early or late writings of Karl Marx; and let's also include the post-modernists, members of that mushroom cloud of European literary writing who seek to rephrase all philosophical questions in seriously unintelligible ways as if to make a fresh point, the point that we must re-discover the questions for ourselves; and more lately, the ethicists and environmentalists have been waxing. If we are shopping around for big ideas, this is a rich heritage once we dust off its books, begin to turn its pages, reinvigorate the lives of some of its great thinkers and re-examine their arguments.

When I arrived at Sydney University, there were two philosophy departments. This was the result of a split in the mid-seventies. I had to make a choice. At the time I didn't know why the split existed. All I knew came from a friend who told me how Liz Grosz, one of the lecturers in the new Department of General Philosophy, for one of her lectures, gave a semiotic analysis of a single page of *The Daily Telegraph*, a Sydney daily tabloid newspaper that rested at the shoddy end of the quality spectrum. Members of the Department of Traditional and Modern Philosophy must have been mortified that philosophy lectures were now incorporating the local morning rag into the teachings of this new Department. But the idea behind the lecture sounded okay to me. Such a semiotic analysis does not look at the words alone but at the inherent power and truth structures within which the words are placed. For me, this makes philosophy more accessible, easier for a newcomer to grasp the issues. At the very least, it was a more sophisticated way of saying we shouldn't believe everything we read in the papers.

Also, when I read the list of subjects offered by the two departments, I saw the logic and reason subjects offered by the Department of Traditional and Modern Philosophy as too arid. I had studied maths in my previous degree and I thought mathematics would be a far better way to deal with all that abstract reasoning and for possibly greater practical benefit if that's what I wanted. So the Department of General Philosophy was an easy choice.

The 1975 split within the Sydney University's philosophy department can be traced as far back as 1965 when students were becoming increasingly more radicalised in the face of many social issues across the world at that time, issues which led many to question the powers running key institutions, highlighted firstly by the demonstrations against our country's involvement in the Vietnam War, and later by the emerging demands of the feminist movement. The source of my knowledge on this period of the department's history is taken from James Franklin's *Corrupting The Youth: A History of Philosophy in Australia*. The title of this book echoes one of the Western world's earliest and greatest philosophers, Socrates, who was sentenced to death for 'corrupting the youth' with his searching, and often embarrassing, style of philosophical questioning.

Before the split, the philosophy department at Sydney University faced a whole series of challenges to its power, including a call for changes in the way lecturers were appointed, and calls for a wider range of subjects to be taught amounting almost to a change in the very definition of philosophy. For example, many were agitating for the introduction of subjects on political and sexual oppression. The establishment, let's define them as being on the conservative side of politics, tried to draw lines and while they conceded, for example, that Karl Marx was a prominent thinker of the modern era, they asserted he was not a philosopher. Students, in seeking these changes, argued with authorities through both formal and nonformal channels, took strike action, and were committed to ongoing disruption for as long as was required to effect change. The result was that, in 1975, the two separate entities, the Department of Traditional and Modern Philosophy and the Department of General Philosophy were formed.

This was the study environment I entered upon my enrolment in 1980. I soon learned that ideological division was a key factor in how many of our philosophers related to each other, that and a fervent commitment to their own splinter position. The situation was reminiscent of scenes of the Monty Python movie *Life of Brian* that satirised British left wing politics in the seventies. It was very close to that: truly a time when there was so much talk and activity but very little clear direction.

Regarding feminism, I had a vague understanding that our society was governed in a very paternal, top-down, power-based, often unfeeling manner, let's call it dictated by a masculine rationality, and that there was room for what we may call a more feminine approach, one more inclusive, more consensus-based, one where decision-makers listened more and didn't just do all the talking. It was a different rationality which many of the post-War generation, including myself, were reaching for. Perhaps it was enhanced by the Cold War environment. However, the feminist movement divided in so many ways on the question of how to achieve a better world based on more attention to a feminine rationality. And some were so harsh, they could best be described as ultra-masculine! The challenges to power were happening everywhere. This was the situation as I was introduced to taiji where my teacher spoke of gaining strength through softness, a very contrarian idea at the time, but one which still has a lot to offer the world. We only need to think of the power of water, one of the softest substances in nature but, at the same time, one of the strongest. My heart was with the feminist cause, but I felt disturbed with some of the anger and militancy of the movement. At that time, I only sensed that modern human society had a more fundamental misalignment than the feminist issue. Over time I find we have a greater struggle with our underlying metaphysical position which once resolved may see many other aspects of society come into better alignment, including feminism-related issues.

For my psychology major, I simply sought to meet course requirements. Very quickly, it didn't appeal to me. Before I enrolled, I imagined psychology to be about the workings of the mind and possible access to its many treasures. What I found was that Sydney University was a bastion of behaviourism, essentially the theory that the human being was a machine whose behaviour could be predicted if we knew the underlying parameters, and this was the line of research which dominated the department. One friend of mine majoring in social work seemed to do a lot of subjects in abnormal psychology, and while I even sat in some of her lectures with her, it never resonated with me. It was like early twentieth century freakshow material.

I did one subject on the psychology of perception with a particular focus on visual perception. I recall how the research in this area was being used to develop machines, for example, address recognition machines for postal services, and there was still a lot of doubt in the early eighties whether such a task was too complex for non-human machines. Obviously there has been much progress since that time. But studying this subject helped me very little in dealing with my own shortsightedness, except perhaps for stimulating me to want better vision that did, over time, come to me.

For my elective philosophy subjects, I was attracted to those linked to the history of philosophy. I enjoyed reading around the lives of the philosophers, from the Pre-socratics up to those of the present day. I struggled with political philosophy and ideology subjects. It was as if, even as a thought experiment, I felt constrained and uncomfortable accepting the assumptions upon which such conversations were based. Perhaps it came down to mastering the abstract language of politics and its dichotomies that was often too dizzying for me.

When we talk about class struggle in Australia it is such an abstract discussion compared to circumstances in other countries. I only realised this later when I was in Manchester in the year 2000. I was talking with a cabbie, and I suddenly realised how this fellow would never shift out of the economic role he was locked into, and he was resigned to be there for life, spending all that he earned simply to maintain his position, with all his seething anger, and for the first time I saw how the class struggle was so much more real in Britain compared to anything I have seen in my home country.

Against this, some philosophers just shone brightly. One worth mentioning is anarchist, Paul Feyerabrand, a man who validated many of my own suspicions about science. His key idea was that science is not the methodical and rational study of our world we were taught in school because there is, in fact, no universal methodology. It does lead us to ask why we revere science how we often do. Feyerabend claims that a close look at history reveals that scientific revolutions and moments of great progress were not due to a predefined scientific method, but often the result of trickery, subterfuge, rhetoric and even showmanship. The biggest example is Galileo's theory of heliocentrism. As a result, Feyerabend's thesis that the most accurate description of scientific method is that 'anything goes', or more formally: epistemological anarchism.

In the course of my undergraduate philosophy studies, I also gravitated towards the existentialist stream of subjects that, in turn, opened me to a new world of literature with existentialist themes and that helped me better understand life in the twentieth century. This line of study led back to the phenomenology of Edmund Husserl and the metaphysics of

Martin Heidegger. What I now notice from my chosen philosophy electives was that I preferred more narrative and reference to the life as it is lived over simple ideas for their own sake.

I was further encouraged in my approach to my casual job at the RSL Club after reading about the great Cambridge philosopher and major figure in twentieth century philosophy of language, Ludwig Wittgenstein. He advocated to his students that, after philosophy classes, they should seek out a menial job, such as working at the counter at Woolworths, where they can test out their philosophical theories and observe human nature in a real life situation. Going even further, he claimed there was no future for the professional philosopher! Despite being the author of one the key philosophical works of the 20th century (*Philosophical Investigations*), Wittgenstein is said to have worked as a gardener in a Benedictine monastery, as a schoolteacher in the Austrian mountains, and as an orderly in a London hospital.

I also enjoyed my anthropology study. I concluded early that the people in this field were mostly adventurers who went out into the world, claiming to study and describe new cultures and societies, and dressing their obligatory reports up with some theoretical analysis. As in our discussion of the perils of breaking down the taiji form into pieces, a la wanting to know what's inside an egg without breaking its shell, I had strong reservations about people who sit outside a society and think that they can know what is going on inside. I am more comfortable that our practice of phenomenology is underpinned by direct experience.

At times, during my studies, I announced I would make a great urban anthropologist. I trace my lifelong interest in corporate cultures back to my anthropology studies. I am endlessly fascinated by how organisations and large corporations function and achieve results. It also helped me better understand my previous experience at BHP, at that time the largest private employer in Australia. And it prepared me for work in government.

One anthropologist who didn't even go out into the world to do his fieldwork was the California-based anthropologist, Carlos Castaneda. He was once hailed as one of the grandfathers of the New Age movement based on his stories of meeting a Yacqui shaman, Don Juan, who taught him the art of sorcery. Castaneda's work was an acclaimed success even though he had supposedly broken the golden rule of anthropology which was to observe and not participate in the community being studied. After he had written some worldwide so-called 'nonfiction' bestsellers of his experiences with Don Juan, it was discovered that the work was fiction and that he had carried out all of his research in his university library to write his works. Some people say his work, regardless of his deception, carries many valuable universals truths and insights.

As Martin Heidegger would express it, my undergraduate study was simple a way of being, which I fully experienced as my life in other areas expanded. Knowledge is itself a way of being, and it was authentic in that I had chosen to be in this situation rather than feeling a victim of circumstance. Once we settle into that state of being, we ask a different type of why, not so much with being with a small b, but we can spend more time on our engagement with Being with the large B. And this was where my taiji was able to flourish.

13 Honours

By my third year at Sydney University, I had a good rhythm going in my new life in Sydney. I looked forward to my weekly lecture schedule, though reading about new philosophers, their lives and ideas often left me feeling drowsy. Getting to the end of a chapter of some texts without falling asleep was often a victory. My biggest motivation was to get my assignments written and handed in on time, a ritualistic struggle for most students.

My two weekend shifts as a glassie each week gave me enough money to live on. With a fun circle of friends, I got to enjoy Sydney's cultural life: seeing bands play live; meeting up with friends in pubs and bars; drinking too much at student parties and then straggling home in the early hours of the morning. Meanwhile, in the tiny though leafy backyard of my semi-detached student house in Chippendale, I assiduously did my taiji exercise routine early each morning. But my university studies and my growing taiji interest never really intersected. They remained separate worlds.

One Saturday afternoon, during a quiet moment in the acupressure clinic, at that time held at the back of the Uniting Church Hall in Canterbury, Simon pulled out an issue of *Scientific American* and showed me an article by George Gale. It was called *The Anthropic Principle*. This principle proposed that the universe has the properties we observe today because, if its earlier properties had been much different, we would not be here as observers now. The simplest example to demonstrate this principle is the distance between the sun and the earth. If the earth was further away from the sun than it is now, then we would freeze, while if it was much closer we would burn. So it is not mere coincidence that the distance of 149.6 million kilometres from the sun is just right. The paper led on to a discussion of the proposal that there are many possible worlds that could exist, but our world is the best of all possible worlds. This theory can be traced back to a seventeenth century German philosopher, Gottfried Wilhelm Leibniz.

Simon said that this idea fits in with the Daoist idea of universal balance, that everything is in its right place, though many people do not see this is so or have forgotten it. Too many are working to repair a world that doesn't need repairing. I had never sat down with Simon and discussed with him what I was studying in my course at university. Although one day I did mention, in passing, I was looking for a topic for my honours thesis. I guess that comment prompted him to dig up this opportunity. He suggested I propose a comparison between Daoist philosophy and the ideas contained in the article he had shown me.

Eventually I formulated a plan to write a paper of comparative philosophy. The particular comparison would be between Leibniz's claim that we live in the best of all possible worlds and the Daoist proposition that this world we live in is the perfect balance of yin and yang. My aim was to show that these two propositions amounted to the same thing even though they were formulated within very different traditions. The intended title was *Tai Chi and the Best of All Possible Worlds*. Most honours theses require a single supervisor but I was told I would need two supervisors for this style of paper.

At first, I was slow to move. We had a Leibniz specialist in our Department but the thought of finding a supervisor for a comparative study of east and west philosophy would be a challenge. I had no idea where to start. However, things do have a way of working out. In my second year at uni, I lived in a share house with an architect. He had studied architecture under Dr Adrian Snodgrass at the University of Sydney who was recognised as an expert in Asian Architecture. Dr Snodgrass gained this knowledge through twenty years of travel around Asia after he graduated. Architecture routinely takes into account social, cultural and even philosophical influences, and Dr Snodgrass had a personal interest in the philosophies of the places where he had travelled. So I contacted him to see if he was willing to supervise my honours thesis. Soon I had my two co-supervisors.

Meeting Dr Snodgrass in his office for the first time, I faced a wizened man with a white beard, piercing eyes, and a wry grin. He smiled a lot and the conversation was relaxed, often meandering. He shared a few anecdotes about his travels through Asia. He told me how during his stay in Korea, he took part in breakfasts consisting of bowls of chopped garlic and ginseng. He lived in a northern suburb of Sydney. He may have been a keen architect but he reckoned he was a lazy gardener letting the trees and plants in his garden grow wild, irritating many of his neighbours, citizens who liked very orderly yards and gardens. However, he said he always had the last laugh because when it was time for the dogs in the area to die they came to lose themselves in his dense, dark jungle.

I met with Dr Snodgrass monthly to update him on my research. These meetings often drifted into general conversations about philosophy. He explained to me that he had studied Buddhism and Daoism in detail. He was also well-versed in Platonic philosophy which helped to guide my research in ways that did not seem available within the philosophy department. For example, he introduced me to the medieval philosopher, Nicolas of Cusa, one of the first Western philosophers since Plato to propose the theory of the coincidence of opposites.

At one of our meetings, as we were deep in conversation, I felt this electric current blasting my third eye, like electro-convulsive therapy. It seemed to be arcing from his third eye. As Dr Snodgrass continued to speak, unaware of the effect he was having, the buzzing went on for about five minutes. Doing taiji for a few years, I mixed with people who were hyper-sensitive to so-called energies around people. Not an easy subject to discuss with people outside your school so it was best to keep stories of such experiences to oneself. Perhaps with that in mind, I didn't react. I just stayed in the conversation, trying to focus on his words as this ceaseless buzzing was going on in my third eye. Eventually the meeting finished and I left, with the whole experience undiscussed, not knowing what Dr Snodgrass made of it. I felt very light, like walking on a cloud, in a different world. It was the most intense psychic experience that had ever happened to me up to that point in my education.

That same evening, we had a taiji class at the Gym and arriving early I was sitting downstairs when Simon also arrived. There were few other people around, and I wanted to share what had happened to me, but felt uncomfortable raising the subject directly with him.

So I just blurted out: 'What does taiji say about the third eye?'

Simon was soft with his words, as he looked into my eyes. Rather than any electric shock, I felt a soothing, as if he understood what I had experienced.

'The third eye is connected to the pineal gland which is the physical manifestation of the unseen centrepoint.'

Simon's use of the term 'centrepoint' referred to the dan tian. This explanation resonated with his teaching about the hormonal system, which Western medicine views as governed by the glands in the brain, whereas Chinese medicine sees the kidneys as the key gland in governing hormonal systems in the body. The hormonal glands in the brain are again a reflection of what is happening in other parts of the body. Recently, much research is being conducted into a set of tissues located in the intestinal area, which some describe as an invisible second brain. The clinical name is the 'mesentery' and it is now being considered as responsible for more and more functions in the body than were previously known.

Simon was never one to talk openly about what nonphysical energy he was feeling at any particular time, unlike what his students sometimes were prone to do. But we all felt he was finely tuned to everything that was happening around him. And it was moments like this, after feeling so soothed by a conversation with him, that led me and my fellow students to constantly wonder about the depth of his knowledge and experience when it came to energy, and how he could deal with all of those energy interactions while keeping such clear physical focus.

My other supervisor, Lloyd Reinhardt, of Canadian background and with a raspy gravelly voice, could be best described as a professional philosopher. While he worked in the Department of General Philosophy, he was more of a traditional and modern philosopher than one of those breakaway types. I do note that he edited a book of dialogues between the two philosophy factions so we could call him a consensus man. He presented undergraduate courses on the progression of modern philosophy, from Hobbes to the modern day. So he was the obvious go-to person for my thesis on Leibniz.

I recall one of his tutorials (held in his office) where we were talking about material and essentials, and he took us through the thought exercise of imagining a boat which undergoes regular repairs where every plank is replaced over time. But the boat keeps the same name, so the question is whether it is the same boat or not?

I also recall another discussion he led one day, of Arabs on camels traveling across the desert who played chess on an imaginary chess board, calling out their moves to each other, and with time to recall the location of each piece on the board as they engage in their long journey.

This leads us to ask the question about where the game was actually being played? Thought experiments like this may sharpen our minds, but they did not lead me to an any clearer understanding of the relationship between the physical and nonphysical. They only reinforced my view of philosophy as a professional activity.

The movie *Searching for Bobby Fischer* about chess prodigy, Josh Waitzkin, who incidentally went on to become a taiji pushing hands champion and author, illustrated just how a key to high level chess playing was the understanding of how much it was a game played in the mind.

At the start of the year, Reinhardt agreed to be my supervisor. I am not sure how it happened, but I astutely managed to slip through the cracks of the system. He went on sabbatical leave for six months not returning till two months before my thesis was due to be handed in. After meeting him early in the year, the next time I recall talking with him was some time in the last semester. I admit I could have engaged better with him or another person within the Department as I stood to receive a great deal of guidance on the project. But I just wanted to research my pet subject of taiji and it felt so free for me to go my own way. Mind maps, networking skills, presentation skills and project management skills were not part of my vocabulary at that time. However, as mentioned, I did consult regularly with Dr Snodgrass so I wasn't a totally rogue scholar.

Reinhardt was determined to have the last say. Following is an excerpt from his assessment:

> 'McGowan shows a persistent tendency to confuse logic and metaphysics.... If I had been in contact with McGowan from the beginning of the year, I would have advised him against this sort of project; so he would have had to do it with someone else or done something different. As things were, I had my first meeting with him in September, when he had already done a lot of work on Chinese thought. I could hardly refuse to co-operate at that point.'

I took his comment that I confused metaphysics and logic as his way of saying that he was not keen on cross-cultural comparisons, and would have preferred if I had stayed totally within the Western philosophical tradition, as its method was based on assertion and argument and logic, whereas much of Asian philosophy is based on pronouncement and development of ideas through resonance rather than logic alone.

Peculiarly, he also commented that he doubted my ability to satisfactorily research Chinese philosophy if I couldn't read Chinese and had to depend on translation, whereas Leibniz wrote mainly in Latin, though also in German and French, and all his work has been translated into English. But he could not see the logical inconsistency in his comments about Chinese. Such a comment again highlights the mood of the times, on how the bastion of rationality as we knew it was under siege. But I had not entered this project to break down any barriers. I was genuinely interested in spending time researching taiji and the Daoist philosophy underlying it and seeking to relate it to my own tradition.

While I invested hundreds of hours throughout the year both in the library and at my desk researching sources for my work, the final task of typing a clean draft of over forty pages of cross-cultural philosophical argument and discussion with detailed footnotes and complete bibliography stretched me to my limit.

This was the era before word processors and I had only recently taught myself to type. My final draft was a collection of 15,000 words with numerous spelling mistakes, many unintentionally joined words which I manually had to seperate with the stroke of a pen, missing footnote annotations which also needed to be penned in by hand at the last minute, a split bibliography between Western and Chinese sources whose irregularity was noted by my second co-supervisor in his final report, and all of that was before I began the flow of my argument and the overall structure of the paper.

I received a second class honours pass and I was happy with that. Our Prime Minister at the time, Malcolm Fraser, had also gained a second class honours in his studies and he went on to become Prime Minister of Australia. I was also comforted by a fellow student at the time who always aimed high. She quoted a favourite GK Chesterton saying: 'if a thing is worth doing, it's worth doing badly'.

The result is one thing, but the journey was another. As a journey of discovery, I had a fantastic year. My way of being for that whole year involved milking the library for all references to Daoism philosophy. This introduced me to so many great works and was a wonderful survey of both the history of Daoism and taiji which none of my fellow taiji students would ever have the time to research. I also discovered the landmark Joseph Needham collection *Science and Civilisation in China* which opened up a whole new world on so many new fronts.

Likewise I discovered so much about Leibniz, and was fascinated by how the collection of commentaries on Leibniz had grown continuously almost since the founding of Sydney University in the late 1800s. I also made the remarkable discovery about the nature of Leibniz's links with China which I will explore in the next chapter. The subject of Leibniz, including his design of the world's first computer, his arguments with Isaac Newton, his connection with Jesuit missionaries in China, and his written proposal to the Emperor of China to establish a world religion, has become a life-long interest of mine that continues to grow.

When I was visiting Kiev twenty years later on a work mission, dining one evening in a very quiet restaurant, an American businessman was sitting across from me. We began chatting and the conversation turned to the subject of Leibniz. He told me that he had previously researched Leibniz and his extensive contact with Russian Czar, Peter the Great: three face-to-face meetings and a voluminous correspondence between them. I admitted that I could not recall having ever read about this aspect of Leibniz, while he said he had never heard of Leibniz's links to China.

To lodge my thesis on time created much angst. I rented a golf ball typewriter from a shop in North Sydney for the weekend before the thesis was due. On the Monday morning, I had to return it to the store before rushing into uni with three softcover-bound copies of my thesis under my arm. As I was lodging them, I met a fellow student who would go on to win the University Medal that year for his first class honours thesis on some obscure point of Marxist theory. His copies were hardcover-bound, gold embossed, and professionally printed and I really felt like one of those awkward outsider kids in one of those bubble-gum American frat movies.

But this had been a year well worth living: I had brought together taiji, my hobby, and my formal academic study in a type of alchemy which few could understand. I had little consideration for the future except I knew I had not lost my passion for taiji after looking at it more closely, and that I may need to find alternative ways to improve my mind than become a professional philosopher.

14 Leibniz

My honours thesis enriched my understanding of taiji in many ways. As it turned out, Leibniz was the best of all possible philosophers I could have chosen for a comparative study with taiji. I was thrilled to discover he had been in regular correspondence with Jesuit missionaries in China about Chinese language, religion and philosophy and they had even sent back translated extracts from the *Yi Jing*. I got to track the first arrival of the taiji concept into Europe.

To survey the phenomenon of Daoist philosophy with any clarity requires a very steady eye. My observation is that a person of Chinese background sees Daoism differently compared to a person of non-Chinese background. We may call this the result of environmental influence. Depending on their age, the former is more likely to be influenced by either their state education against the old superstitious ways, or through their more recent direct exposure to the ornate ceremony and ever flowery language of Daoist religion which they may today equate with the philosophy. The person of non-Chinese background, mostly unfamiliar with the religious culture of China, will often see the philosophy through their own ingrained social conceptions of nature and freedom and so on.

The original people who practised Daoism never called themselves Daoists. They just reveled in life without thinking much about it: using the ordinary things in life to taste its greatness. For them, everybody is connected to the source of all things and so could be expected to look after themselves. Life was more about maintaining this focus on the connection to the great source such that their life was a steady unfolding of actionless action. Sometimes, with a headstrong urge to do, people veered off the main road of dao, but their by-road would eventually meet up again with the main road so that was really no problem. These people had no label. It was others looking at them who labeled them Daoists.

Over time, Daoists seperated the mystery of life from otherwise mundane aspects of living and soon Daoism settled into a form of mysticism. There are many tales of Daoists who could perform amazing feats. Originally, such feats were simply a spinoff of their study of the dao, not an end in themselves. This is where yin and yang theory was introduced and became a justification for division. They forgot that yin and yang are two aspects of the one force, in a way that yin and yang become two fundamental forces which appear difficult to unite without the intervention of the mystic.

The next step was Daoist religion, where the divisions became more rigid. We see a colourful proliferation of rituals, saints, deities, artworks and texts which are all valid expressions of the original dao but which are also accompanied by a snowball of ignorance where judgements and pronouncements are often made, many employing false assumptions about the original nature of the universe.

The essence of Daoist metaphysics can be expressed very simply. We have an infinite and undifferentiated energy of the universe that can be seen from two perspectives: firstly, its original creative aspect and, secondly, its receptive aspect (nonphysical and physical). All beings carry the original creative aspect and, as manifestations, reflect all that is in their own unique physical perspective. The rest becomes detail: the manifested world is the most colourful display of yin and yang forces. We can become very lost in the yin-yang detail if we overlook our link with the original creative source.

Before we investigate Leibniz's metaphysics, it is helpful to include some words about his life more generally. In this short space, I can only list some of Lebniz's wide range of interests. While he worked in the field of law, he had a personal interest in languages, mathematics, biology, medicine, geology, physics, politics, ethics and navigation. He is introduced in the high school mathematics syllabus as the joint independent founder of integration and differentiation (co-founded by Isaac Newton).

There is a series of correspondence between Leibniz and Newton, where they argued about theories of absolute versus relative space. While Newton argued for absolute space, Leibniz put forward his subtle arguments for relative space. I do wonder whether Leibniz was actually a forerunner to Albert Einstein's theory of relativity and the era when Einsteinian physics would replace Newtonian physics.

It should be noted that Leibniz never sat down and wrote a comprehensive account of his philosophical system. We obtain his ideas and arguments from pamphlets he prepared and from correspondence with fellow philosophers, scientists and students.

Leibniz's metaphysical system is considered to be one of the first organic philosophies in the Western world. This metaphysics is underpinned by a perfect God, while the world consists of numerous substances which Leibniz called monads, where a monad cannot be divided into parts. Each monad perceives the universe in its own unique way and the closer the monad's perspective is to God's will determine that monad's level of perfection. Leibniz denies that one monad can have an effect on another monad as they are essentially windowless.

When asked how they all share the same world, Leibniz introduced the concept of the 'pre-established harmony' between all monads, there since the beginning of time. Joseph Needham proposed that Leibniz obtained his organic ideas from Chinese philosophy. Others have argued that it is merely evidence of a pre-established harmony between his and the Chinese ideas. They argue that Leibniz had his idea of monads from an early age. His first reference to China was made in his writings when he was twenty years old. However his father died when he was seven and his father being a teacher, left his son a library full of philosophy and history books which he eagerly read, so the argument is that he was well read and had formed a lot of ideas before his first contact with China.

Extending Leibniz's view of the physical world in its totality, Leibniz proposes that there are an infinite number of worlds, each with its own qualities. The world that we live in, Lebniz declared is the best of all possible worlds. He claims that this world may also be described as that with the greatest variety and the greatest order.

Leibniz developed one of the first automatic counters which some consider to be the first computer. It was based on a binary system of counting. It is this adoption of a binary counting system which opened up his interest with the Chinese philosophy of the *Yi Jing*. Noticing that the hexagrams of the *Yi Jing* are based on a series of lines depicted as either light or dark (yang or yin) he felt that Chinese metaphysics had a basis similar to his own, and at one stage he wrote a letter to the

Emperor of China suggesting that they could develop a world religion with a rational basis.

My thesis was focused on a comparison limited to the metaphysical systems of the Daoists and of Leibniz. I did not have time to explore the historical, diplomatic, religious and political dimensions of Leibniz's engagement with Chinese culture. There was so much more room for exploration. Since the time of my thesis in 1983, there has been a proliferation of publications on this aspect of Leibniz's work. Up until the time before my thesis, Leibniz's interest in China was largely overlooked. I am so pleased that Simon had the foresight into the opportunity, seeing way ahead on so many levels, when I was simply focused on getting by at university from semester to semester.

Regarding the history of the term 'taiji', we in the West share the vague assumption that the term has had currency in Chinese philosophy for maybe thousands of years. It is true that the term was used in the *Yi Jing* where it is written: 'In the Yi (Jing), there is the taiji. This generates the two primary forces. The two primary forces generate the four images. The four images generate the eight trigrams...'

However, there is little general use of the term again until the time of the Neo-Confucianist philosopher, Zhou Dunyi (1017-1073), when he presented the Diagram of the Supreme Ultimate (Taijitu) as part of his metaphysical system. The taiji symbol emerged at about this time. The more specific term of taiji quan can be traced to Wang Zongue around 1700. I have dealt elsewhere with the rise in popularity of taiji quan and the associated taiji image and philosophy at the start of the twentieth century.

The taiji concept was introduced by Zhou Dunyi as part of a conscious effort to provide a metaphysical underpinning to Confucian social philosophy. Again, this was convenient as a buffer to Buddhist religion which was growing in popularity at that time. Buddhism had a strong metaphysical basis and had a lot less to say about social rules and regulations. Evidence indicates that the taiji diagram was borrowed from a volume in the Daoist Canon called 'Diagram of the Taiji which Antedates Heaven', a volume which contained a preface by Emperor Hsuan Tsung (715-755).

As far as my research indicates, the following extract from a letter by Leibniz to a friend in Europe, marks the introduction of the taiji to Western thinking:

> 'According to the Chinese, the Li or the Taikie is the One par excellance, pure goodness without admixture, a being completely simple and good, the principle which formed Heaven and Earth; it is supreme truth and strength in itself, yet not confined to itself; and in order to manifest itself, created all things. It is the source of purity, virtue and charity. The creation of all things is its proper science, and all perfections come from its essence and its nature. This principle comprehends all the ways and the laws of reason (external as well as internal to itself), by which it disposes of all in its time without ever ceasing to act or create. It can be assumed that the Li, Taikie, or Xangti is an intelligent nature which sees all, knows all and can do all. Now the Chinese could not without contradiction attribute such great things to a nature which they believed to be without any capacities, without life, without consciousness, without intelligence and without wisdom.'

Leibniz stood out very strongly in his day for his interest in cross-cultural exchange. While he may have been naive and ignorant in many matters relating to both China and Russia, he was bold enough to step outside his own Western tradition seeking what he claimed was the universal good. He felt that the West could particularly learn more about ethics from cultures in the East. With China, he proposed to the leaders both in Europe and in China for more systematic cultural and intellectual exchange, what he called a 'commerce of light'.

Before the Catholic Church could give their assent to such exchange, there were two issues which they needed to address: the first was the question of whether the Chinese had a word for God. Leibniz argued that they in fact did have suitable words, for at least three thousand years. These words were 'shangdi tian' and 'taiji': the second issue was whether the Chinese rites for the dead were civil rites or religious rites. If they were deemed to be religious rites then they would be considered idolatrous and not compatible with Christianity. The debate was framed as the question of 'accommodation': whether the Church could accommodate the ancient Chinese words and practices if Chinese were to become Christians.

In 1710, the Pope declared they would not be accomodating to the Chinese, and he proscribed the Church in China. Emperor Kanghsi, likewise, declared the Jesuit's unwelcome there too. And, for the next hundred years or so, the European interest in Chinese philosophy was kept alive by a very small number of individuals, mostly friends of the returned Jesuit scholars.

15 Meditation

In this chapter, I intend to explore meditation as a phenomenon in the modern world. Meditation is of more than passing interest. It goes back at least to the time of Pythagoras where we learn how his students meditated on various geometrical shapes. However, it is worth investigating meditation in its contemporary context rather than in some bygone golden age.

In practising phenomenology, we focus more on description than explanation. We takes things as they are and reflect descriptively on how they present themselves to us. Significant patterns of relationship and explanation will find their own way to the surface as a secondary part of this process.

As part of my Catholic education, I received a detailed introduction to prayer from an early age, including stories about how how Jesus prayed, how many of the saints and of course how our teachers and ordinary people prayed. Prayer was accessible at any place and any time. I do remember observing that people seemed busy while praying, like they were doing all the talking, and not much listening.

Most Catholic children receive rosary beads at some time in the course of their education, most often when they receive the sacrament of Confirmation. The specific design of rosary beads is a large ring of five sets of ten beads with each decade being separated by one large bead. This ring of beads is linked to a smaller strand that holds one large, three small, and one large bead and at the end of that a crucifix. There are a series of images and items for contemplation for different days. Some people can become attached to their rosary beads and wear them around their neck. We can easily conjure the image of a lone person seated or kneeling in an otherwise empty church, and they are holding each bead of their rosary and rubbing it with thumb and forefinger till their prayer is said before they move on to the next bead, interspersing sets of Hail Mary's, Glory Be's, and Our Father's.

When in infants school, I took prayer seriously, saying my morning prayers as soon as I woke up and my evening prayers before I went to sleep. In high school, the lessons on prayer continued. Meditation was not on the curriculum. However, one day, the subject did come up in a science class. Our science teacher, who we saw as probably our most switched on of all our teachers when it came to knowing what was happening in pop culture and wider society, commented that meditation is a helpful thing to learn but he reckoned we shouldn't have to pay a lot of money to learn it.

Sadly some people sell meditation as more than the tool that it is, they embellish it and drape it in mystery because, in that way, it can become a lucrative source of social status and income for them. The greatest value of meditation is in its regular daily application. It is not intended as a substitute for other activities in life. It is a simple method to teach and to learn. My first direct experience of meditation, in my late teens, was via the previously mentioned book, *Three Magic Words*.

Meditation as a word emanates a type of neutrality, a sort of independence of being, and a seeming capacity to accommodate any number of new users of the word for what we may define as their mind-focused practice. The word has eluded domination by any one group over the decades, or possibly over centuries, and it has done this through yielding to all who seek to use it. Meditation equally accommodates practitioners who embrace techniques from the East or the West, the mainstream or the esoteric, the new or the old. As a word, it retains much of its original meaning and has not become tired or bogged down with excessive ideology. And so we may even say it has been a good advertisement for itself.

However, I do sometimes wonder if my earliest impressions of meditation were tainted by late sixties and early seventies images of yogis, usually male, with long grey hair, moustaches and beards, people sometimes barely dressed, sometimes in flowing robes, garlanded by flowers and surrounded by followers, sitting with their arms crossed and eyes closed purportedly at the doorstep of nirvana. The image of Maharishi Mahesh Yogi easily comes to mind but I also recall other more austere versions of the yogi who may, for example, be sitting on beds of nails to demonstrate the powers of mind over matter. But this was the impression of an outsider, one with a Christian school education that placed much value on the virtue of prayer.

That same above-mentioned Maharishi Mahesh Yogi developed and taught a form of meditation known as Transcendental Meditation (TM) that could be easily integrated into the Western lifestyle for the benefits of relaxation, stress reduction and self development. TM is one of the most thoroughly researched techniques of meditation in the world today. I recall how in the 1970s in Australia TM gained a lot of attention as its advocates here were seeking to prove that if the square root of one per cent of a population practised daily meditation over time then that community would collectively experience its benefits. Though the evidence of this is still disputed, it is a noble vision, a new age take on the socialist dream.

One great value of TM is its simplicity and its ease. So simple that in 2013 Jerry Seinfield told a story at a David Lynch Foundation dinner where he said he started practising TM in 1972 and went on to enjoy a successful career as we all know. However, when introducing his son to the practice forty years later, he discovered that he had not been doing his TM right all that time, and from then on he went on to receive more benefits. Seinfield uses the image of doing TM as like charging your cell phone to full each day so you don't have that feeling of running on empty.

Many people today would argue that because different activities are described with different names they must be different. But I have come to discover that prayer and meditation have a lot in common, particularly in their aims. But being part of very different traditions, with their different methods and approaches, of course they will carry different names. But each of them are seeking the same thing.

Taiji is a meditation tool with a spiral-like approach that can suit anyone from those who simply want relaxation and relief from stress all the way through to seekers of how to achieve the very best that is humanly possible in their life.

For new students, we introduce taiji as a dynamic form of meditation. The postures are based on circular motion, and as we move, we focus our mind on the quietness at the centre of that circular motion. We follow the movement as it goes up and down, left and right, forwards and backwards, much as we do in life. We soon find our centre of gravity and are able to relax as we experience this movement. This makes taiji a very realistic form of exercise for we develop the skill to calm ourselves while engaged in our inevitable daily activities. We find the quietness inside the motion. There is a saying in taiji: 'stillness in stillness is not the true stillness, stillness in movement is the real stillness'. So this is how in the first instance we introduce yin and yang to our students and suggest how we may harness its interplay to improve their life experience.

Once a person is comfortable with the postures and they are flowing well, there is a lot to ponder within the postures and with the traditional imagery associated with them as previously explained in the chapter on taiji form. We use this form to go beyond the form, after which we can return to the form to see it in a fresh light. We also employ circular breathing which draws us into the centre.

Taiji, therefore, is a meditation on the co-ordination of our mind, body and breath. What tires many people. and ages them faster, is the disharmony between these three zones of being. When they are working against each other, we generate resistance. Taiji coaches us to let the different parts of our being come back to their natural harmony. We use our body to go beyond our body, our mind to go beyond our mind and our breath to go beyond our breath so we are immersed in the energy of our nonphysical being. From there we come back to the body as it is, the breath as it is, and the mind as it is, and through this we can refresh and feel clearer about ourselves.

The highest level of taiji is where the person practising it becomes so immersed that the line between meditation and daily life becomes so fine that life becomes a type of meditation, a dynamic meditation, where we are relaxed and flexible and revel in each moment of our life. Our life experience becomes smoother, problems attract their solutions a lot more effortlessly, and we are more friction-free as we move from one moment to the next. At the same time, meditation becomes a wonderful experience, without boundaries, without limit and something that can be practised anywhere and anytime.

When people discover meditation and how it seems to lighten their life, it is natural that they would want to share it with others close to them. In efforts to do this, it is amusing that the argument for doing meditation is so often framed in scientific terms. We only need to do a quick survey of youtube clips on introductions to meditation to see how so many advocates quickly turn to scientific research to validate their meditation technique, with reference to experts in the fields of physiology, neurology, psychology who produce results that suggest meditation may be of some benefit.

Taiji has been the subject of high level research at such mainstream educational institutions as The Harvard Medical School. Such researchers are investigating areas such as general wellbeing, preventative medicine, drug-free pain control and faster recovery times. Much of what science will do in the future is to validate what the taiji teaching has been saying for centuries.

The benefits of meditation is very much in the doing. It is far from a one-dimensional activity that will conform to the gaze of science. Here we may use the analogy of a garden bed where rather than add one ingredient, it may be better to focus on building up the soil, the humus, where the plants are able to grow better and can more easily adjust to weather conditions because they can draw more or less of whatever they need from the ground. Too much attention on each individual plant and ignoring the soil context may take more energy for less results.

In this work, I have spared you that scientific analysis which can become so dry. To appeal to science can often means that there is a mismatch of beliefs and one is trying too hard to win over the other. In my experience as a taiji teacher, the best policy is to let people come to us. This is an indicator that they are ready to learn, that they feel the need for meditation, and that they have done their homework. Once they begin learning taiji, or meditation, they will be able to discover for themselves whether it is helping them or not. If they have questions, then hopefully we can help them find the answers.

A good meditation routine is also a valuable foundation for a person to develop a viable metaphysic to help them navigate life. We have seen in our lifetimes, a move away from organised religion with their ready-made codes of living. Those old forms do not seem to have been delivering as well today as in the past. Organised religions may be able to adjust to meet the needs of today's and tomorrow's members, but there is a growing community of people who wish to explore their own path in their own way without conflict with others who do the same. They want their own compass and meditation is a very useful tool in that case.

16 Teaching

Simon encouraged his students to seek out opportunities to teach taiji. His view was that when a student comes to a taiji class they are, in fact, not even at the learning stage. They are still unlearning. They can be unlearning bad habits of physical posture and movement, unnatural breathing patterns and unhelpful mental habits such as not being able to stand freely in the present moment. It is only when a person goes out to teach that they really start learning taiji. The teaching process helps them to clarify what to do and what not to do. Taiji is only about leading a horse to the water, it's nothing to do with making it drink.

I am reluctant to use the word 'teacher' these days. The word seems loaded with a relationship of power between teacher and student. When he was demonstrating the two person taiji exercise Pushing Hands where we learn to flow with another person, not fighting and not running away, Simon often used the words: 'I owe you nothing and you owe me nothing'. This really was a statement of about how the centre of the motion saw the two people interacting and obligation played no part in this. The spirit is one where when we help others, we are helping ourselves, and when we help ourselves, we are shaping to help others. The best teaching environments carry the same spirit.

Anybody who has taught anything face to face knows that teaching is an immersive activity. During the process, we cannot separate teacher and student. It is a dynamic wholeness. For one who has not taught they can imagine that there is a line between the teacher at the front and student in the classroom, but that line disappears as the learning process takes over.

It is the same with taiji. As we move together, we harmonise in very deep ways. We begin to feel what other people around us are feeling, be it the joy of expansion or the pain and discomfort of resistance. It is almost as if ideas drift from one mind to another seeking out a home. The process is that we all direct our minds into the centre of the motion and that centre of the group expresses itself with a powerful momentum which each student chooses to either go along with or not.

The task of the teacher in such a taiji situation is to guide the group even as the group expresses its own character and its own flow. In fact, we get to experience exactly what the great philosophers like Lao Zi talk about when they speak of how leaders best lead when they are following. This is something that we cannot learn from a book. The essence of taiji is non-resistance and the single effort of the leader of the group cannot fight the group, it can only go along with it. And by doing that, they keep pointing out the direction. Nothing more. This is where we are learning at a very deep level how to apply our taiji maxim: use mind and not force.

In my first year at university in the Gym when I was learning the long form, Simon gave his attention to the beginners while he asked me to lead the form to the students who started the previous term. While I enjoyed the idea of sharing, I felt the responsibility, it was like I was holding the fort while Simon was occupied with the beginners. But to step up to the role of the one leading the group, I felt the immediate increase of the group energy. I was intimately linked to the energy of the whole group and was being asked to lead under Simon's more detached guidance.

Simon once told us of how he learned taiji from his teacher. His teacher taught very few people, less than ten. He channeled his taiji realisation into his healing clinic. Simon would go around to his teacher's house and do the form while his teacher was engaged in other activities around the home. At the beginning, Simon wondered whether his teacher had forgotten about him. But through his comments at the end of the session, the teacher let Simon know that he was closely aware of all that Simon was experiencing while he was doing the exercise. The best taiji is an energy flow, it is not the performance of artistically correct taiji postures alone.

In teaching the postures, Simon was always walking that fine line of teaching as holistically as possible while meeting the needs and expectations of the students. His style was to keep moving and even talk a lot while demonstrating the form, whether it was calling out the names of the postures or giving more general advice like keeping our knees bent and looking straight ahead. I enjoyed this holistic approach, I could always go home and practise what I had learned and this sharpened my focus on what the missing pieces were.

I continued to teach my own taiji classes in various locations around Sydney. I felt I had something valuable to share with others. I found it most convenient to operate through the local adult education networks. These colleges did all the administrative work, and I simply taught in particular time slots at particular locations. I attracted many different students, people with busy jobs, other people were referred by their doctors, some had once studied a little taiji years before and wanted to revisit it. Others were searching for answers to deep philosophical questions. I recall one student who attended a workshop was a pole dancer but had a persistent bad back and thought taiji would help her.

In the steps of my teacher, my intention was to use these classes to introduce taiji to the community and then to offer more serious students the opportunity to continue away from the school so we could spend more time on the long form and examine how to incorporate taiji into our daily life, and perhaps even teach others. This worked okay for a few years. However, at that time, seeing how the internet was emerging, I decided to develop a correspondence course on the taiji idea. This was in consultation with Simon who was then semi-retired on the South Coast of NSW. He reminded me of the qi gong correspondence course he did when he was in high school.

In our classes, we could see the trend of how people were often too busy to learn the long form of 128 postures. In response, we had shortened the form to an introductory set of five flowings plus the first two cycles of 27 postures. Going further, Simon was of the strong opinion that the most important aspect of taiji was the idea. And the taiji form was simply a vehicle for this idea. And so with this in mind, with my writing skills and my knowledge of the history of taiji, I developed the idea of opposite meditation as a focus for meditation practice and a tool for softening some of the harsh one-sided thinking and attitudes which seemed to be taking influence in wider society.

I developed a set of notes and exercises for the course and a one day workshop to introduce the subject. I also wrote several articles some of which were published, the biggest success was with the premium health magazine *Wellbeing*. I have included this article as an appendix to this book. A few smaller articles were published in other new age magazines.

The idea of opposite meditation is that everything has its opposite. It begins with a widely accepted scientific law: Newton's Third Law of Motion which states that: 'in any physical system, for every action there is an equal and opposite reaction'. Life will become a greater and greater accumulation of uncomfortable resistance if we ignore this basic law of science. This is why we recommended students to regularly practise opposite meditation, to learn how to see both sides of a situation and therefore be more holistic in our thoughts and actions. Over the years, in line with our understanding of ourselves as creative beings, we have refined our understanding of our theory of opposites. While understanding the total situation, we engage on the wanted side of any equation, and detach from the unwanted. While we felt there was a lot of benefit to be had through this philosophy, it was certainly not glamorous as we cited examples such as Newton's Third Law of Motion which everyone had learned in early high school. Though you could say we were also into recycling.

As I was developing this course, I received an invitation from my employer to work overseas. I was asked to go and work in Moscow for three years. On the opposite side of the world! This opposite meditation worked so well for me!

I knew, if I was to later teach, how important it would be for me to demonstrate that my philosophy was able to enrich my own life and career. So I shelved my wishes to set up a school in the suburbs. I had my own path to follow and it didn't feel right to simply stay and repeat what I had seen my teacher do. After my return from Moscow, I had a brief stay in Australia before I worked in Africa on a short term mission and then went to work in China for three years.

During my time overseas, I still wanted to share my taiji and found myself writing more about the subject.

After I returned to Australia, I co-operated with the local adult education college in Wollongong and offered introductory taiji courses and also one day workshops. But I noticed that the people were not sticking with it. I wanted to find new ways to express the taiji idea and for me that involved writing more about it.

I've never said no to a person who wanted to learn taiji from me, but I also know that I was not attracting the following that my teacher commanded. I knew that the right thing for me to do was to follow my own path.

17 Health food

I worked as retail store manager in the health food industry for seven years and during this time I learned a lot about about nutrition and health as well as how people engage with health food. This included two years at the previously mentioned Rozelle Health Food Centre. My greatest observation is that all food is beneficial to our body and a 'health food' attitude is as important to us as the health food itself. I also observed how there are times when we will be drawn to certain foods that will be good for our body in more ways than we intellectually understand and it helps for us to know how to go along with our body wisdom when it speaks to us.

The simple label 'health food' can offer much insight into the psychology of the human being in our modern world. Traditionally, the label has been associated with foods that are richer in nutrition rather than poorer. For those in want of that richer nutrition, the term fires the imagination with visions of health and vitality. Yet there are many who yawn at the sight or sound of the phrase. They know how much the words 'health food' have been used and abused over the decades. This is where belief comes in. Food is just food, they may say, you only need to see it from the point of view of our stomach with its low pH (high acid) levels. And sooner or later, somebody will trot out the story of the lumberjack who worked hard for long hours each day at low temperatures and survived on cupboards full of tinned cabbage. Because he had the right attitude. It is a very contested territory, this question of mind over matter.

When we stand back and examine the health of our nation as a whole, we cannot fail to notice the astronomical cost of health care. In Australia in 2016-2017, we spent $180 billion on health and this represented ten per cent of overall economic activity. Given that this cost is rising year by year, I have no doubt we need to investigate health food not just as a lifestyle preference, but as a tool to improve our national productivity. If health, as some claim, is all in the mind, then health food may be a way of administering a healthy attitude.

I want this book to be fresh, with fresh ideas expressed in fresh ways. But I do need to remind readers of the old expression: one ounce of prevention is better than a pound of cure. This is about finding health and keeping it, and getting sickness in its early stages rather than its later stages which requires such intense and costly attention. And there is enough evidence, both scientific and anecdotal, that prevention is better than cure, that healthier eating habits can lead to a healthier person and that to a healthier community.

Before I started infants school, I accompanied my mother on her weekly visit to the local health food store in the main street of Campbelltown, just down from the Post Office. So I was the recipient of some good early imprinting. The walls of the store were lined with shelves holding wooden cupboards with glass panels behind which they kept all the different bulk foods such as flours, grains, nuts, seeds, dried fruits and more. I have vague recollections of the staff in the shop wearing white jackets which gave them a clinical look about them. My mother did a lot of cooking and baking on Saturdays and she bought many of her ingredients from this store. It would be many years before I discovered how such stores were part of such a long tradition which started in the United States in the mid 1800s. Thomas Martindale reputedly opened the first health food store in Philadelphia in 1875 and a lot has happened in the space since that time.

I next recall while I was in high school, there was an amazingly successful marketing campaign by a company called Hunza. Their premise was that all these people in the Hunza Valley, a region that borders China and Pakistan, a high proportion of them lived to at least one hundred years old. Some people claimed their longevity was linked to their diet of natural and unprocessed food and so Hunza promoted their line of products with the suggestion that we could all have such longevity if we ate similar foods. I recall eating my Hunza muesli each morning before school as did my father as he prepared for work. Health food stores stocked many products stamped with the familiar Hunza label.

As we studied taiji and attended the natural medicine clinic on weekends at Simon's place, Simon repeatedly impressed on his students and patients the three pillars of good health: healthy attitude, healthy exercise and healthy food. These three pillars are mutually self-supporting. It was against this background that it made sense for us to open our health food store in Rozelle. It was a logical progression of all that we were doing up to that point. We had a strong team and were enriching our own knowledge and experience of health food to reinforce our taiji teaching and natural healing practice. It was a type of life research.

Our team of eight partners signed a two year lease for a property on Darling Street Rozelle, just behind a pizza shop on the corner. I had recently graduated from University, and had been looking for work in a health food store around Sydney. Before this Rozelle opportunity came up, I had taken the page from the phone book listing all suburban health food stores and had approached each store seeking work, but didn't get an offer. As all other partners had full time work, I was nominated as co-manager with another partner.

I did not claim wages at the Rozelle Health Food Centre, I was doing work for the dole long before it became a government policy. The store for those two years usually broke even once rent was paid, so I was occasionally given a box of food on Saturday afternoons. But I was comfortable with this arrangement, as I was learning all about managing a shop as well as discovering a lot about the health food game.

Turnover did not grow as fast as we hoped. There were a few new trends in the mid-eighties which challenged our financial viability. In the seventies, health food stores were the prime source of bulk food for the new trend towards health. Also share houses, especially student share houses in the name of frugality, would turn to health food stores to buy their staples. Before this time, supermarkets generally had a small speciality area dedicated to the health food shopper. But it was at this time that they began to take on more and more health food lines. Also, traditional loyalties were giving way to market forces. Before that time, Blackmore's, a herb and vitamin company founded in the 1930s, had a policy of supplying their herbs, vitamins and cosmetics to health food stores only. They provided strong support to the industry. But in the mid-eighties they changed their policies and decided to deal with pharmacies. They installed the full range of products into a pharmacy store around the corner from our shop. Before that we only stocked the Blackmore's products that our customers wanted. We could always take special orders for the fortnightly delivery but we could not afford to carry the whole range.

We decided not to renew the shop lease after two years because of the financial situation and also some of our partners were heading off to other adventures. We disposed of the fittings and distributed the leftover money. It was demanding but I had revelled in these two years so much, I wanted to remember it so I put a few hundred dollars of the money distributed to me to buy a men's dress ring, amethyst stone set in nine carat gold, and I had it made by a jeweller in The Centrepoint Tower in the city as a memento of my precious learning experience.

Once that business closed, I walked into a job in a Vita Health Food Store in King Street in the centre of the city around the corner from the Pitt Street Mall which was being constructed at the time. This new shop was turning over about fifteen times the volume of the Rozelle Health Food Centre but as a store manager the routine was exactly the same, so I really felt like I had landed on my feet. This was a good example of leverage. Working here felt special because in the fifties and sixties my grandfather ran a popular fabric shop only a few dozen metres around the corner in Pitt Street, so I felt some sort of family continuity with my working in the centre of the city.

Manly Palmer Hall in *Adventures in Understanding*, writes about how Daoism in Asia is often the religion associated with the merchant. The merchant, who goes to their shop each day to buy and sell, who is constantly struggling with competitors, wholesalers and the fickle public, they find it beneficial to develop their Daoism in terms of learning to relax and accept the vicissitudes of life, the yin-yang interplays, the joys and disappointments from all the interactions in the course of a day, the feeling that buying and selling is largely a game which becomes a way of being with the hope that the business will provide enough for themselves and their family.

I too found retail to be such a way of being. It was an opportunity to practise what I had learned in taiji. We would go in there fresh each morning, ready to extend our fresh qi through our hands to persons and products alike as we endured the whirlwind of the day returning home to refresh and do it all again the next day.

One aspect of my work that I loved was to discover some great personalities in the US health food industry. They were already old by that time, but their books just kept selling. They continued with what seemed like a fresh message. People like Paul Bragg (1881-1976),

Norman Walker (1886-1985), Herbert Shelton (1895-1985), Adelle Davis (1904-1974) and Ann Wigmore (1909-1994). They were giants in their personal advocacy of health through nutrition and natural foods and supplements and their story is largely untold outside the world of their immediate admirers.

We have had some significant spokespeople in Australia as well. Without entering into the debate of the medical establishment versus the natural health profession, I must mention the tribulations of Dr Archie Kalokerinos who worked in outback indigenous communities and oversaw a reduction in infant mortality rates with the administration of large doses of Vitamin C. Dr Kalokerinos was a highly qualified doctor, having been appointed, amongst others roles, as a Life Fellow of the Royal Society for Health, a Fellow of the International Academy of Preventative Medicine, a member of the New York Academy of Sciences, and in 2000 was awarded the title of Greek Australian of the Century. However, he only ever received a cold shoulder from the medical establishment. He could not even get a letter, let alone an article, to the Australian Medical Journal published. It was rejected on the grounds that his work was not scientific.

In the US, there is also a huge story behind the medical and pharmaceutical industry's powerful resistance to the use of Vitamin E for heart problems despite plentiful evidence. Suppression and obstruction works for a while, but such experiences only bring about a stronger desire for health through natural means which must eventually win out.

There was a generational surge in demand for more attention to cleaner more natural and less processed food. Within the industry, we learned very quickly to withstand attacks from vested interests. Whenever I see a report coming out saying that vitamins or minerals or herbs are of little or no value, I mostly just shrug and wonder to myself who wrote that report and who paid for it. The real health food is part of our evolution and cannot be stopped.

In the Bondi Junction store, trade was busy, though at the end of the 1990s interest rates went really high and retail sales were down across the board, especially in health foods, my employer got out of retail to focus on his wholesale business and so sold the store to new owners. I felt like it was time for a change of career.

119

However, all of the health food knowledge and experience I gathered in those days stays with me today. I have built in so many small yet beneficial steps to my preparing meals. For example, I always keep a jar of Brewer's Yeast in the cupboard and add a spoonful to all soups I cook to enrich the nutritional value of the meal. Brewer's Yeast is rich in B-complex vitamins and minerals.

Ironically it was in the health food store where I learned that healthy eating was not enough in our quest for total health. At the front of the shop, we had a large rack holding all the different brands of bread supplied by small local bread makers. All were wholemeal, some made more rigorously than others, eg with organic or biodynamic ingredients. I recall a customer who came into the shop one day and picked up a loaf and read the ingredients and then turned to me very angrily and asked, 'Do you know that this has got salt in it? How can you sell stuff like this?' This angry customer was so helpful to me in bringing clarity to my understanding of health foods because now I know that a calm and receptive state of mind is so important for good eating, no matter what we are eating.

In conclusion, it pays for us to have confidence in our food choices and to take more time to enjoy the food that we eat. Our body instinctively knows to absorb the best of what we eat and spin away the unwanted. The simplest Daoist prescription for healthy eating I have ever come across consists of the following three steps: a) eat as naturally as possible; b) eat as much of the whole thing as possible; and c) eat as much variety as possible.

18 Chinese language

After five years of practising taiji, and being out of university for two years, I felt the desire to know more about Chinese culture to better place my taiji tradition so I decided to enrol in a course of Chinese Mandarin language at Sydney Technical College. My long term goal was to read the Chinese classic, *Dao De Jing*, in its original. Maybe I finally succumbed to my honours thesis supervisor's criticism about my lack of Chinese language skills.

Studying Chinese language has directly enriched my taiji through a clearer understanding of many of the philosophical concepts expressed in words of the original language. The language has also been a wonderful window into Chinese culture which is a great storehouse of human experience. Another advantage of my language study which I want to highlight in this chapter is the simple benefit of knowing a second language. It is easy to overlook, but a second language helps us to see outside our normal world in a way that we come to see ourselves more clearly. Some people may speak a number of languages without ever considering this, but I see it as a great tool for us in the modern world.

After four years of classes on Tuesday nights, I gained a certificate in Chinese Mandarin, which more reflected the time I had invested than the rewards I had reaped. I was still at an elementary stage of conversation. However, I was well grounded in the basics of the language. Chinese spoken language has four tones and it is helpful to get these tones clear early on, which I was able to do. I also used some quiet time early in the day in my health food shop to practice writing Chinese characters. Al Huang, a taiji teacher in the United States, taught calligraphy as part of his taiji workshops. Apart from meditating of the components of each Chinese character, such exercises at the physical level serve as a flowing experience. The brush is held by the hand, but the energy of the whole body drives the hand.

I recall a conversation with one of my language teachers at Sydney Tech College who did a double commerce and arts degree at Sydney University studying Chinese as a major, and he told me how he was disappointed with how little Chinese he could speak at the end of his degree course. He remedied that by going down to Darling Harbour when Chinese merchant ships arrived and striking up conversations with the sailors, and he says that's where his language skills really began to develop.

I always dreamed of one day writing my own translation of the *Dao De Jing*. That dream is still alive. Though I notice these days that online we can see hundreds of translations of this work available. It is not necessary to do our own translation, but it can be a rewarding activity. Over the years, I have dabbled in translation of some of the popular taiji treatises written over the centuries. I also attended a classical Chinese translation class at the University of Sydney where I was taken through some classical Chinese texts of Meng Zi and Zhuang Zi. This was only ever an introduction course for me. But it allowed me to dabble more efficiently with translation at home.

Before I focus on a case study highlighting the issues of translation in Chinese, I want to draw the reader's attention to a colourful phenomenon of Chinese language, the four character saying, *chéngyǔ* (成语), an idiomatic expression that often tells a story, captures a moment of human experience in a rich and concise way and is often able to be read at a number of levels. One simple example is qíhǔnánxià (骑虎难下). It means- it is easy to get on the tiger but hard to get off. It can be applied to many situations in life, consider for example any addiction. I am also reminded of this phrase when a former politician is described as suffering from 'relevance deprivation syndrome'. We may also see a tattoo in this light. There are many *chéngyǔ* and they can be such gems of human experience. As the following discussion will reveal, *chéngyǔ* are open to much interpretation, especially in translation.

One of the simplest and most well known taiji treatises is the previously-mentioned Yang Cheng Fu's *Ten Essential Points of Taiji*. I have included my translation at Appendix Two. While this is very short, it truly highlights issues involved in translating Chinese, I have taken the first of Yang's ten points to share some insight into the pleasures of such translation. It is a phrase of only four characters: 虚灵顶劲 (xūlíngdǐngjìn). To support the case for treading carefully in translation, Lee Fife's online work *Yang Chenfu's Taijiquan Theory: Ten Essential Points* lists the following translations of this four character phrase.

1. Effortlessly, the jin reaches the head top (Ben Lo and collaborators)
2. An intangible and lively energy lifts the crown of the head (Louis Swaim)
3. The spirit of vitality reaches to the top of the head (Robert Smith)
4. The energy at the top of the head should be light and sensitive (Doug Wile)
5. Open the energy at the crown of the head (also Doug Wile)
6. Empty dexterity's top energy (Guttmann)
7. The spirit, or shen, reaches to the top of the head (Jou Tsung Hwa)
8. The spine and head are held straight by strength, which is guided by the mind (T. Y. Pang)
9. Empty, lively, head-top jin (Barbara Davis)
10. The mind should be light and spacious, having the quality of perpetual alertness so that the spirit will rise and the inner energy emanate through the top of the head. (Wolfe Lowenthal)
11. Empty, lively, pushing up, and energetic (Jerry Karin)
12. Empty Neck; Raise Spirit (Sam Masich)
13. Insubstantial jin to lead the crown upward (Yang Jwing-Ming)

The problem with taiji translations often goes back to the authors, many who wrote in a compact style so that students could remember entire strings of phrases. And we have the added step of translation into a different language.

Having my elementary Chinese skills, I am less prone to taking words on face value. I am more likely to focus on what a person is trying to say. And of course my interpretation of this may change over time, but that's okay.

There are many benefits in knowing a second language, particularly in the way it allows us insight into both the people and the culture behind the language. Again the cause of many international conflicts in the past have come down to communication, and I see a greater role for our strategy of using our mind more and force less even at the international level, not just at the interpersonal level.

John G Bennett (1897-1994) was a British mathematician and scientist with a strong interest in meditation and Sufi philosophy. In his book *Witness* he described how he took up the study of Turkish language towards the end of World War One and it was at that time that he realised how much language dominates our thought patterns. He concluded very quickly that, though they were both Europeans, English speakers cannot think the same as Turkish speakers. Our language format of subject and predicate strongly influences our deep-seated subject-predicate logic. In the Turkish root language, he says, there is no predicate form. They don't even have sentences, but more like single word complexes that express a speaker's feeling about a situation.

I mention this here, because I have been thinking about the role of language in the shaping of our world view for a long time. We at least need to be aware of how language may be shaping and colouring our world. I studied French and Latin in high school but wasn't aware at the time, language at that point in my education was more about word substitution. Globalisation was once a project largely carried out at the individual level, now it has become a collective phenomenon and we need to have better communication skills if it is ever to roll out successfully.

When I started studying Chinese, I thought Chinese was so difficult for an English-speaker to learn. It was different in so many ways. I made slow progress. It was a typical case of taking lots of risks and using opportunities to strike up conversations even if they don't get far. As they say, the sooner we make our first thousand mistakes the sooner we can learn. But in 1997 when I was invited to work in Russia, I began Russian language classes. Now here was a complex language. It is like Old English with its complexity of cases and declensions. It was only at that time, that I felt this enormous appreciation for Chinese language and its elegant simplicity: it has no tenses; no verb conjugations; no male and female endings; no cases; no irregular cases, no strong and weak nouns; agreements; subjunctives, singulars and plurals declensions etc.

New features of Chinese language such as measure words, particles, word order rules are more like mathematical rules which allow you to set the context and conditions before the main business is discussed. It adheres undeviatingly to its conventions, eg matters of time and place where the larger always comes before the smaller.

As I took various runs at my Chinese language studies, I joked with people that Chinese kept throwing me back to my English language and literature. It was the contrasting experience of another language which helped me to see my English language in a new light over and over. It also helps me to see my Australian culture in a new light where I know more clearly what I do like and know what I don't like. It is easy to think that studying a second language is about the other, but that second language enriches our self. The self and the other are inextricably connected. When we look at the other, we see ourselves more clearly. We are not sacrificing ourselves by looking at other languages and other cultures. This is living taiji: yin for yang and yang for yin.

My ongoing interest in both metaphysics and language prompts me to pay special attention to wider social examples where language issues influence our wider society.

In 1990, I joined the Department of Immigration which I will talk about in more detail in another chapter. Immigration law in Australia underwent a huge change in 1989. There was a new focus on definitions because the courts were clogged up with challenges to decisions made under the pre-1989 legislation. Many of these challenges were based on the meaning of words used in that legislation. For example, what does the phrase 'compassionate and compelling' really mean or what does 'genuine' mean in the context of a spousal relationship. The single word 'refugee' carries millions of words of clarification in guide books and court case decisions and yet the term is as contentious as ever. Monolinguists are less likely to appreciate the issues involved. They are more likely to use power or force to resolve issues instead of 'thinking them through'.

Rubing, my wife, has taught Chinese over many years at all levels, from introductory up to university level. She is systematic and methodical in her teaching, intuitively harnessing the students' natural enthusiasm to learn a new language. The closer the language teaching comes to examination processes, the more of a labour the language study becomes. And the more resistance creeps in. We also have parents who seek to impose their language heritage onto their children and children can resist this. Such children may not drop out of class but they passively resist. After observing Rubing's teaching experience and hearing many stories, I have come to the conclusion that the best ingredient to a successful language learning program is to study in a spirit of fun, to enjoy it and to see it as an adventure. This is very different to the way I had foreign language introduced to me in high school in the seventies.

As we stand on the brink of the widespread introduction of new technology which will allow word for word translation to be done a lot quicker than ever before, the issue of cross-cultural communication remains a challenge for all of us. We will still need those broader communication skills which go way beyond language itself.

I have a lovely example of the pitfalls of word for word translation across languages which I have enjoyed sharing with friends over the years. When in Russia, I sought out a Russian language teacher soon after arriving. I had found her through an ad in *The Moscow Times*, a local English language newspaper. Her name was Svetlana. The classes were to be held at her apartment in a southern suburb of Moscow. Winter had arrived and it was cold and snowing heavily. I made it to the door of her apartment, with my heavy coat, scarf, hat and boots. Svetlana welcome me in and said, 'You get undressed and I will be in that room.' She pointed to a room and then disappeared into it. I did a double take, hoping I was sure that I had read the ad in the paper right. I eventually took off my coat, my scarf, hat and boots and meekly entered into what was the kitchen where Svetlana was sitting as she asked me what took me so long. The issue was that the Russian word for taking off your coat, раздеваться, is the same as the word for undress, so I had a Russian-speaker using her English the best way she knew how, but it came across with a slightly different meaning to a native English speaker.

Finally, do consider locating a copy of Lao Zi's *Dao De Jing* and reading it. There are many translations available online. Find a copy you feel comfortable to read. To gain most benefit, I suggest that you read it when you are relaxed and in a happy mood, not when you're feeling disturbed or upset.

19 Visits to China

While in high school, I would occasionally visit my Uncle Peter and Aunty Camille's home, a few streets away, for dinner. They enjoyed a good discussion over a meal on all sorts of subjects. When the two of them disagreed, whether it be about a family matter or a question of food or musical taste, my very Mancunian Uncle Peter would often yield to Camille's argument and turn to me and quip: 'Patrick, marry a woman and become a philosopher.' This was one of Peter's strategy for finding peace with the world, of how to be with another.

I studied philosophy first. I had been in a few relationships in my twenties. I was advised by Mark Gruner, a well-known local numerologist, whom I met in a shopping centre in Sydney when I was about twenty-one, not to marry till I was at least thirty. Was this advice or a prediction? I only followed what felt right to me, and that's how I got to be with my wife, Rubing, at the marriage registry office in Sydney in my thirtieth year. Rubing was born in Singapore but grew up in mainland China. She came to Australia five years before we were married. Her father was a journalist and supported Communism so he returned with his family to China from Singapore in the fifties and remained there. We married within a day or two of the Berlin Wall falling down which we all noted as an auspicious rapprochement between East and West.

One of Rubing's hobbies over many years has been Chinese painting. Chinese watercolour painting is a refined art where a few deft brush strokes in a few colours can produce striking images of objects. When I first met her, Rubing had several favourite subjects: prawns, flowers, chickens and horses. She could paint a horse with such ease, a horse that looked so filled with vitality, with all the attributes of a prize winner, a horse so noble and with such a fine coat. And yet one day when I took her out to a horse ranch to do some actual horse-riding, she was so uncomfortable and didn't want to go near a real horse. Apart from the smell of the manure in the yard, there was the dusty coat and the dry hair of the mane and the sounds of it walking and its reservation of the right to be an animal with its own mind. I'm sure she much preferred the abstract and it really took some coaxing for her to join us on the ride.

This shift from the abstract to the real was similar to my experience of China. I had read a lot about China, learned some language, had a few Chinese friends, been to lots of Chinese restaurants where I learned not to have a seat facing the kitchen etc, and I praised many aspects of Chinese culture. And after that I went there. I made three trips to China in the first five years of our marriage.

The first trip was a short ten day visit to Beijing to meet Rubing's mother and the rest of her family. It was July and the weather was hot. This was a time when the majority of vehicles on the road were bicycles. There were very few cars. I recall how we wanted to go a few kilometres to a metro station and we decided the easiest way there would be to hail a bicycle rickshaw. An old man pulled up and invited us to sit in each of the seats behind him. His face was showing the strains of the hot day and he never twitched when we told him the destination.

He slowly pedalled hard to build up speed and when he had his momentum up he relaxed and wanted to chat. We told him our story. And he told us he was saving money to send his child overseas to study. From my perspective, there was a gap so huge between a man earning a few Chinese dollars per hour and a child needing thousands of US dollars to study overseas. It was a gap that left this hero totally undaunted. I was quickly reminded that each person has a right to their own dream.

Another memorable moment from this first visit was the day that Ruby's friend lent us her driver for the day. While on the road I badly needed to use the toilet. While toilet availability is now at international standards, at that time clean public toilets were hard to find. Public spaces were owned by all and owned by none. Our quick thinking driver took me to a shopping centre, newly built, parked the car and lead me down to the basement, opened a door and in we went. But to my dismay, there was no light. It was pitch black in the bowels of the building and I was absolutely bursting to empty, so luckily my driver was a smoker and he lent me his lighter. He kindly offered to come in and hold the lighter while I did my business, but I politely declined his offer.

Our second trip was to visit more relatives and stay in Beijing for the Chinese New Year. This time we caught an overnight ferry from Hong Kong to Xiamen where Rubing's sister and her family lives. The ferry was very old world, it was a people mover, no thought was given to the joys of cruising, even if this did sound like an exotic way to approach mainland China. One detail I recall about this trip was that our cabin, smelly and unventilated, was that the lock on the door was broken, so when we did eventually go up to the deck or to the kiosk for dinner or fresh air, we had to surrender ourselves to the fate of the journey. I recall the sense of elation on this visit to China that would last ten weeks. In the late afternoon, I recall being on the deck with clear weather, we were sailing eastwards, and with the moon being full, it was so brilliant to see the sun, an orange ball on the horizon set at the rear of the ferry as the moon rose at the front, sun and moon in opposition, a foreshadowing of the experience of the contrasting moments to come.

As we were disembarking the next morning, right near the exit, I saw a man offering to change foreign currency, something illegal in China at that time, and standing right next to him was a policemen staring off into the distance. So, I again quickly learned that when in another culture, we do need to learn to manage contradiction, otherwise moments of contrast can be hard to understand. This was the time we entered China with two video tapes of Rubing's favourite show *Bugs Bunny* that she wanted to show to the younger members of her family. At the time there was a campaign against pornography so all tapes crossing the border had to be examined so we were delayed about an hour at customs till the officers could confirm our *Bugs Bunny* story.

We finally made it to Rubing's sister's house. Rushi and her husband, Yongji, welcomed us with a meal. Yongji, who was a master of hospitality due to his position within a tourist and trading company, explained to me right away that food was the central object in Chinese culture and to eat Chinese food is to study Chinese culture. He said he would go further and insist that food is a god in the eyes of the Chinese people and so they treat it very reverently. And so I was a little surprised the next day when we were on the ferry from Xiamen to the small island of Gulangyu and sitting across from us were a young couple eating apples, and when the male finished his apple he just threw it on the floor while the girl decided to spit out a mouthful of her apple. But I was getting the hang of being in China, as Mao taught a whole generation of Chinese, we need to embrace contradiction because he reckoned the key to life lies in contradiction itself, like the contradiction that the Communist Party is atheist but an image of its greatest member, Mao Zhidong, hangs in most taxis because he is considered a god with supernatural powers. I don't agree with Mao's ideas on contradiction and find it better to resolve any contradictions as quickly as possible for both health and peace of mind. But we will return to this subject later.

That visit, in the name of taiji research, I made it a point to visit the White Cloud Taoist Monastery in Beijing. It was said to have been visited by Zhang San Feng, and was famous as a source of Taoism propagation, and so as I got closer to where the temple was supposed to be and I saw right behind it a huge smoke stack spewing out white smoke, I knew there and then the Taoist masters, where ever they were, must have had a great sense of humour.

It was easy for me to wake up early every morning and go to a local park and stroll for a while before choosing a semi-private space to my taiji moving meditation. I was just another person in the park enjoying the morning air. There were often large groups doing taiji which I could have joined if I wanted to. But while I always enjoyed seeing them in action I felt more comfortable doing my taiji alone.

My association of taiji with Chinese culture also came into clearer focus. In the parks in the morning, while there were many taiji groups dotting the parks, different people were involved in so many activities: dancing; walking; running; singing; calisthenics; mahjong; calligraphy; card games; yum cha; walking the dog and so on. I was even warned to avoid the money changers in such places because they were like magicians and would expertly rob me blind right under my nose if I gave them the chance.

Our third visit to China was a short stop over in Beijing on our first flight to Europe, another eye-opening experience. By this time, I felt like an old China hand and planned my excursions each day getting out and enjoying the sights of Beijing even as Rubing stayed at home with her mother who was now getting old and never went outside.

I was moved by my visit on the outskirts of Beijing to Yuan Ming Yuan (Gardens of Perfect Brightness), the site where, in 1860 during the Second Opium War, foreign armies sacked and looted China's imperial treasures. It's still a scar in the Chinese memory and serves the government as a relatively recent reminder of the dangers of dealing with hostile foreign powers.

I know it is a separate issue, but when I saw this I was reminded of the Boxer Rebellion in 1899-1901 and the tragedy of the Chinese martial art nationalists who believe so much in their own qi power and they could repel the Eight Foreign Armies. They stood bravely directing the qi from their hands at the enemy but so many were mercilessly shot down where they stood. This was an important moment in the history of taiji as well. Simon, my teacher, would always say if you want to kill someone, it would be better to go and buy a gun. Taiji is about something very different to this.

As I share my account of my discovery of Chinese culture, I wonder about our country's relationship with China. Each generation of Australians consider China and Chinese culture as new stars on the horizon, a new phenomenon. We so easily forget our past. I recently discovered that the ships that brought the convicts out to Australia in the First Fleet in 1788 dropped the prisoners and soldiers off and then sailed directly to Canton where they backloaded their ships with tea and other goods for the return voyage to England. There is also evidence of pre-1788 trading between Chinese sailors and our indigenous people. So our relationship with China goes back many hundreds of years at least, and yet we seem to so easily forget this history, almost as if we deny any relationship with the other so that we are driven to re-discover it again each generation for ourselves.

As an example of the endless unfolding discovery of the detail about China, it was only this year that I learned that our use of the word China comes to us from the Persian word Cin, the land of Cin, which is drawn from the name of the famous first Emperor of China, Qin Shihuang (259BC to 210BC), whose tomb still remains unopened in the outskirts of the ancient capital of Xi'An.

20 Public service

Moving through my high school years, I was often impressed by how many of my school colleagues were so clear about their intended careers. I had colleagues who went straight to teacher's college from school and they have worked as teachers ever since. Other colleagues walked into law and engineering studies, quickly found their place and continued to flourish as they accumulated more and more experience. I never felt any such sense of direction and I never experienced any such feeling of purpose when it came to career. I meandered along, making abstract decisions about where to work, not feeling any passion for any particular position. I had some sort of wanting but it was far more undefined.

As mentioned in an earlier chapter, when I was twenty and was considering leaving my traineeship at the steelworks, I felt drawn to the idea of studying taiji as a hobby. With very little research into the subject, it was like I saw a light and thought to myself, that's something I could really enjoy! It wasn't a career, but it was a wonderful way to invest my time.

With taiji, came opportunities in the health food business and I embraced them. After our health food store in Rozelle closed down, I settled into the role of retail health manager with its routine shop hours. I worked for a company named Health Minders. They were a wholesaler who also owned a series of Vita Health retail stores around Sydney.

But retail was a precarious game at that time. One winter, I took a one week break down the far south coast of NSW and saw how cheap land was down there, about $20,000 for a standard quarter acre block. Getting back to Sydney, I made an appointment with the loans manager at my local Commonwealth Bank and he didn't even bother to exert enough energy to laugh at my request. He just said that being a retail manager was a high risk occupation and so would not help me to receive a loan. He promptly told me he was busy and asked me to leave.

I worked for Health Minders for five years, with stints in their City, Maroubra and Bondi Junction stores. In 1990, they decided to focus on wholesale and get out of retail so they sold the Vita Health chain. The new owners had little direct experience with the health food industry. They were just investors. As interest rates climbed, I had the feeling the business would not survive. So as a type of insurance policy, I did a public service entrance exam. Some months later I was offered a job in the Department of Immigration which was good timing because my health food store closed one month after I left. The Department of Immigration has changed its name with almost every successive government so I will use this as the generic name covering the immigration portfolio ie visas and migration and settlement whatever its formal name may have been over the decades.

Apart from my assessment of the poor prospects for that health food store, now being married, I had devised a plan to buy a home and so calculated I needed a steady job, maybe for ten years, to pay for it. I still had no burning passion for any particular type of work, but the immigration workplace slowly grew on me and I ended up staying there for nineteen years. My wish to share what I strongly believed to be the best taiji in Australia took a second place but that was not such a bad thing.

Joining the Department of Immigration was a blessing in many ways. To say that this portfolio was highly political may make it sound like a liability. However, the fact was that every time a problem arose, the government sought to quickly solve that problem by throwing more money at it. So I was able to advance through the ranks with great ease. When the tide rises, all boats rise with it.

In the early nineties, there was a strong government focus on increased training for workers across the Australian workforce. This phenomenon was partly connected with the wages accord between government and unions where unions agreed to forego larger pay rises on the condition that a higher percentage of an organisation's budget was spent directly on staff training. So all of a sudden, after working in retail for about seven years with zero formal training, I was being sent on client service courses that would last up to five days. We had lots of training, ranging from conflict resolution to enhanced computer skills to stress management.

I also received a lot of valuable management training. Again, it was an irony that I was the manager of four staff in a retail store but I had no formal management training. I could do no more than define myself as an apprentice to Simon for the two years we had the health store in Rozelle, but that was all. I recall one day when there was tension between two of the female staff in the Bondi Junction shop and word had got back to the national manager. His simple instruction over the phone to me was to fix it by the end of the week or he'd sack us all. Take this as a window into Australian management in the late eighties.

Up until the eighties, the politics in Australia was shaped around the power of the unions versus the union-breakers. But in a classic case of creating their own resistance, the anti-union forces were so focused on their enemy, they had lost sight of good management practices. There are many examples of bad management decisions which have lead to enormous wastes of resources at national and local levels. And yet the same people continue to say that the only way to lift the nation's productivity is by getting people to work harder. But I had learned early in my work life that whenever there was trouble it was usually two sided, for we all now know about Newton's third law of motion, for every action there is an equal and opposite reaction.

All of this experience stimulated within me a strong wish to discover what constituted good management. In the public service, moving from section to section, I worked for many different supervisors and managers. A lot were outstanding people, thorough professionals. They were technically sound, they treated people well and were often able to harness the best in their staff. I soon came to the conclusion that there was a nexus between the taiji idea and good management. It was a particular book *In Search of Excellence* by Tom Peters which crystallised this idea for me. He classified management issues as being either hard or soft. The hard issues were mostly capital, financial and equipment. But Peters pointed out that it was often the soft issues, things like interpersonal skills, managing perceptions, self-management and corporate culture where better productivity gains in a company were most likely to occur. So I slowly learned to speak the language of management and it became my hobby to study up on the subject and find out what were the leading edge theories of management. Of course, most corporate warrior-scholars have access to bookshops full of the latest management trends and fads where subjects covered include oriental classics such as Sun Zi's *Art of War* and *The 36 Strategies*. But without a core, all these trends and ideas and tools don't hold. They fade very quickly. I found that with my core of taiji understanding, I was able to consolidate many of these new ideas and incorporate them into my workplace behaviour.

After five years in the Department, I was sent on a government-sponsored public sector management training course where I gained a Diploma in Management. Held in a series of blocks of four week classes plus workplace-based assignments, this course crystallised a lot of ideas I was processing in my efforts to discover how to better incorporate taiji into my daily working life.

As the Department of Immigration held the responsibility for implementing multicultural policy, all of our staff were well versed in multicultural speak. For me, it came down to recognising the value of diversity. Being an island continent far from many of the world's great centres of culture, mainstream Australia has traditionally tended to be inward looking and wary of outsiders. But with the explosion in communications and travel, Australia was unavoidably becoming more exposed to overseas influences. While the speed of change brought on by these factors has caused some resistance, we do generally see the value of diversity. Diversity has to be the watchword in promoting any multicultural policy. From the grass roots level of team dynamics, managers who can harness the diverse talents and experience of members of the team will get better results. Their team will be more productive. At the national level, Australians who speak foreign languages and understand foreign cultures and customs are more likely to unlock and develop trade opportunities. To acknowledge and accept diversity is a case of how simply by letting go of resistance, which can often be costly in itself, we can achieve much better results.

More generally, as a society, for a long time we have held strong beliefs in the use of force particularly in the need to force people to achieve certain outcomes, though now we are seeing that this can also be very costly and inefficient. Maybe this was part of the learning from the fall of communism. While the socialist dream may be a wonderful dream to hold, we can't force it onto people. It simply won't stick. We are now discovering that the best way forward is for people to manage themselves more, to become better self-managers. So that if what authorities consider to be good for people, people will adopt those practices under their own steam. So a leader's role is becoming more to establish a better environment where people will make better choices.

Again, as a community, we are evolving to use mind more and force it less. It is time for us to make this shift in our personal lives too.

This brings us to the question of culture. I mentioned that since my undergraduate days in anthropology, I have taken a close interest in corporate cultures. The Department of Immigration employed about 6,000 people when I worked there. With so many individuals holding so many different beliefs and values, there would be some days when I would sit at my desk and wonder how anything gets done in a day in an organisation like this. But it was consistently meeting the demands of all its stakeholders. Our culture was multiculture, people were our business. We saw through the social and cultural wall to people, always people.

Some very strategic planning was behind this success. The best people were recruited, these people were well inducted and trained to perform their duties, and their performance was continuously reviewed. Something I enjoyed about working in this portfolio was that we felt so connected to the national political agenda. This Department was part of the nation building agenda, which it had been since the end of World War 2, and its work touched with so many other departments from business, welfare to foreign affairs and so on.

Of course, large organisations will from time to time make mistakes. For example, in the mid-2000s after a government inquiry, we were found to have acted improperly and unlawfully for holding a long term permanent resident in detention for an extended period of time and also for having deported an Australian citizen. While suffering severe criticism from some quarters, the outcome was a top up of $50,000,000 to better train management and staff. I underwent an executive management training course from this funding top up.

Being in such a busy, inspiring and challenging workplace over so many years, my taiji served me well as a backup, both in the way of regular physical exercise and also meditation to relax my mind. Knowing how good taiji was and not wanting to let go of it, I continued teaching night classes at a local adult evening college and also did one day workshops several times a term. As a presenter, I was getting lots of good ideas from my workplace which I was translating into my taiji classes and workshops, including how to structure a training course, and how to deal more professionally with students.

It is time for us all to become better self-managers, what ever our status or role in the workplace. Whether we coach ourselves or find a suitable coach or mentor, it's a beneficial for us to take that step. One day, our self-management skills will become our greatest asset.

As to the perennial question of how we best manage contradiction and paradox, taiji can offer us a lot of insight. We need not fear contrast, including differences of opinion. We know how to respect and value diversity. Enforcing conformity will only lead to exhaustion. And then there is still the residual resistance. The key will be forever in the field of self-management after which managing people and other resources becomes so much easier.

21 Seeing the world

In taiji, we say that life is a circular motion and when we put ourselves into the centre of that motion, it will draw to us all the people, times and places we need for our balance and expansion. After being born and bred in the suburbs of Sydney, and with little more than a few short trips overseas to Singapore, Hong Kong, Taiwan and China, the circular motion suddenly took me out into the world in a bigger way than I ever remember imagining. I happily went with it. Over a period of nine years I would work in Russia, Kenya and China. It began with a posting to the Australian Embassy in Moscow starting in August 1998. I was notified one year before so I had time to prepare.

When I think back for clues as to the conditions that contributed to my getting an overseas posting, I don't see any hard striving. If anything, the best that I can say is that I always had an idle curiosity about different people and places around the world. When I was younger, my Uncle Peter would tell me that he could always tell a person who has travelled and I would think to myself that I wanted to be one of those people.

Zooming forward to the mid-2000s as I was living in China, I smiled, with a touch of awe, when a vivid memory came back to me from when I was about sixteen. That was almost thirty years before. At that time, I was an avid listener to the music of super groups of the time. Besides enjoying their music, I loved to read about their lives and their lifestyles. I recall reading how members of some groups essentially lived in five star hotels. I was prompted to imagine, to daydream, what it would be like to live in a five star hotel, not just as a tourist but to actually live there. That memory popped into my head as I was living in the Apartment Tower of the Garden Hotel in Guangzhou, one of the three five star hotels in the city at that time. I was there for three years. This was deemed to be secure accomodation suitable for an Australian-based officer serving overseas. I immediately felt that I had well and truly received the answer to a question I had posed long ago.

But going back to the start of my almost ten years of working overseas, to be notified of my first posting to Moscow was within the range of expectations when I think back to the day I did my public service entrance exam in 1989 while still working in the health food store. I was asked to nominate any particular departments I would like to work in. At the time, I simply wanted steady and reliable work, but since they asked, I identified my preferred departments as either Foreign Affairs or Immigration because I knew that they sent staff overseas and that sounded like a good idea to me.

From when we got married in 1989, Rubing and I always thought that for us to live and work together in China would be a wonderful thing. Towards the end of 1994 we went on a short trip to Europe (with our free stopover in Beijing) and we loved it. Europe with the grandeur of its history and culture opened up to us. So we decided that if I ever applied for a posting, I would firstly nominate European posts before posts in China. As part of the posting process, I was asked to number all my preferred locations in order. However, what I did was to number all European posts as number one. My interpretation of this non-compliance with instructions is that the decision maker said: 'Look! This person has put Moscow as number one. Quick, let's get that off the list!' Moscow was not a heavily sought after post, due to weather, the general post-Soviet living circumstances and its rating as a hardship post at that time. And so Moscow came to me.

The work was demanding, with its long hours, constant struggles and setbacks dealing with old equipment and difficult office accommodation, but that did not dampen what was a fantastic cultural experience away from the office. Being classified as a hardship post we were compensated in various ways, eg an extra week's holiday each year. On my way back to Australia three years later, I had two passports filled with visas and stamps, and I counted that we had been to over 36 countries and some of those countries I had visited several times. This list included countries we had visited for both short holidays and work trips.

Being in such an unfamiliar place as Moscow, life quickly became a series of sharing stories with others, listening to those who had been there longer, and telling others about our own new adventures. I was saturated with stories: from clients, work colleagues, the local newspapers, people I met randomly. I came to accept this torrent of life experience. I kept a box with cuttings of quirky newspaper stories, travel books, tickets, brochures, maps and souvenirs of places I visited, half-finished notebook journals and newsletters, letters and cards etc. My boxes of records kept growing into a disorganised mountain of paper which could only ever point to the richness of the experience we were having. The following words of Lao Zi occasionally came to me:

'The heavy is the root of the light,
the unmoved is the source of all movement.
Thus the Master travels all day
without leaving home.
However splendid the views,
he stays serene within himself.
Why should the lord of the country flit about like a fool?
If you let yourself be blown to and fro,
you lose touch with your root.
If you let restlessness move you,
you lose touch with who you are.'

The Russians say it another way:

'ъ гостях хорошо, а дома лучше;
to travel is good, but home is better'.

Rubing and I regularly checked the *Moscow Times* for events in Moscow. We attended so many classical music and ballet performances, rock concerts, international soccer matches, movies etc etc. But we also kept our eye out for the more quirky events. Early in our posting, we saw a small ad for a pending performance by an experimental musician who made music from various metals taken from aeroplanes. It was a small show to be held in a private apartment. We caught the metro and trudged through the snow to get to there.

About twenty seats were lined up in the loungeroom. As background, the performer, whose name I have long forgotten as I will explain below, had for a long time collected metal parts from planes. As they were all of a different chemistry, each had a different timbre. These many metal pieces, of different heights and shapes, were hanging by wire from the ceiling. He was also interested in shamanistic ritual and he introduced his show with a type of alchemy of fire and ice. He had a large wok with a fire burning inside it and he had collected snow from the street which he placed on a tray above the fire so we saw the interaction of fire and ice. To top it all off, as the place was so crowded with guests and music equipment, I recall the performer wearing nothing but a pair of underpants as he ran from one metal item to the next tapping to produce his music from these metal objects hanging from the ceiling. We later talked with his girlfriend who spoke some English, a woman from Siberia who was a student of shamanism, very trendy at that time. I had certainly never seen any sort of show like that while living in Australia.

This is all from memory. The following night, I prepared a long email describing the performance in detail and sent it to a few friends in Australia but have long since lost that email. So now I only have my raw memory of the event. I tell this story to demonstrate the range of experiences we had to share. We have been to many many unusual and unique gatherings during our stay in Moscow.

In earlier days, diplomats faced travel restrictions as part of their conditions of working in Russia. This was of course reciprocated for Russian diplomatics living in Canberra who needed host country permission to travel beyond fixed distances. We faced no such restrictions and we bought a new car and travelled 30,000 km in the less than three years that we used it. We visited so many galleries and museums, especially former residences of writers, musicians and artists, and former battlefields. We also drove across to the Baltic states and many other regional cities. We enjoyed driving in both the Russian summers and winters.

I was on a high during this posting. I did not take a sick day which I attribute to the way I managed m own health through attitude, exercise and diet. In the warmer months, I went to parks early in the morning to do my taiji on the way to work. With my background in health foods, and let's say health more generally, I quietly observed how others managed their own lives as well. To visit a Western doctor at one of the international clinics was very expensive. I observed much over-servicing of members of the expatriate community. One statistic I heard was that about 30% of the expats had their gall bladder removed while living in Moscow. It was times like this when I was so happy with what amounted to my own form of self health insurance.

After three years in Russia, I can say I had seen a lot more contrast and diversity than if I have stayed in Australia. I could appreciate the different experience of the land and its people, even if I didn't understand it. I just accepted that Russia and the West were on very different wavelengths. We can interpret this in many ways. Some say people of the West are ruled by the head while the Slavic people are ruled by their heart. So they think in different ways. I am reminded of the double headed eagle, the symbol of the Russian state, with all its ambiguities, perhaps as found in nature, whereas the United States, with a different focus, is symbolised by the single eagle, the one that flies above all of God's creatures.

Returning to Australia, I took a job in our office at Sydney Airport. This meant shift work, early starts and late finishes. I managed this for two years before I was off to China, but my stay at the airport was broken in 2002 with a nine week short term mission to Nairobi office to help in dealing with some heavy caseloads. Again I used my weekends there to explore as much as I could including a safari to the Serengeti National Park, the Rift Valley and a weekend in Mombassa.

Some say that nothing is as magical as your first overseas posting. But at least you are more prepared for subsequent postings. In 2003, I was fortunate to be posted to Guangzhou for three years. My introduction to China and Chinese culture was largely via my wife who grew up in northern China. Now I would be working in southern China, a whole new world, a whole new step in my China experience.

Work in the office was again busy as we faced cutbacks in Australia-based staff numbers even as we saw the caseload growing. We worked long days and at times, overtime on weekends, to both complete projects and also to reply to information requests from offices in Australia at any time of night or day. It is no secret that fraud was an issue at this post. We were required to make evidence-based decisions on many claims made by our visa applicants. In administering the migration caseload, I faced both contrived marriages and contrived divorces. It became a type of game, this question of whether something was true or false. I was dealing with a culture that placed a different interpretation on the concept of truth. Again this was a contemplation on the nature of truth as we, government officers, sought truthful answers to all of our questions. I still challenge people to honestly answer the question, if they were given the choice, of whether they would prefer to know the truth or to be happy, which would they choose?

Curious about this human dilemma of true versus false, I adopted the hobby of shopping for jade. Collecting fine jade in China is a tradition that goes back many thousands of years and it is arguably a central element of Chinese culture. Jade is a metaphor for many things in this life. One aspect I grew to enjoy was its subtle metaphoric equivalence to truth and sincerity. We have so many stories about people presenting substitutes of jade as the real thing. And it has been endlessly rewarding to explore this subject: it sharpens our own senses; we better appreciate people with the necessary skill and experience to make such judgements; and we become a lot more watchful in our dealings with others. We very quickly look beyond jade and turn our incessantly questioning mind to other fields such as friendship, art, and even government. Here is a hobby that is like a bellows, that keeps giving with new insights into human understanding and always new stories. One day I hope to conduct an in-depth phenomenological analysis of this thing we call jade.

Apart from doing taiji each morning in the luscious gardens of the Garden Hotel, I also used my evenings to maintain some journals which became profound formative experiences for me. The first was the financial journal process called *Your Money or Your Life* by Joe Dominguez and Vicki Robin which really helps the reader through a series of exercises to develop a clearer relationship with money, something I had never really thought much about before that time. They also introduced me to the concept of financial independence, something that occurs when income from non-employment related sources equals your expenses, a very valuable moment especially for an intending writer. I also began an amazing journal process as taught by Ira Progroff called *At A Journal Workshop, Writing to access the power of the unconscious and evoke creative ability.* This is a writing process with really life changing results as we tune into deeper parts of ourselves and understand ourselves as part of a greater being. I felt so rich in time and energy in China to achieve all that I did.

While in Guangzhou, I travelled regularly for both work purposes and also for leisure. In each of the places I lived, I occasionally wrote newsletters of my travels for family and friends in Australia.

I discovered that there were five sacred Daoist mountains in China: Songshan; Taishan; Huashan; North Hengshan; and South Hengshan. I wondered whether I could visit and climb them all and decided to use my leave breaks to make the climbs. I climb the last of them, Songshan, near the famous Shaolin Temple on an icy, snow-covered day in December 2006 when I was on my way back to Australia at the end of my posting. I still marvel that people have been trekking to these locations for over 2000 years and I am part of that tradition.

On our training course prior to departure overseas, we were advised that there were several key indicators of whether a person would have a happy posting overseas. The biggest indicator of an unhappy posting was going just for the money. I went for the experience and adventure and to do my work well and it all turned out well for me.

146

22 Returning home

Hexagram 53 of the *Yi Jing* is *Jian* 漸, meaning *Gradual Progress*. It is an image of a tree growing on a mountain. Internally, we have the image of the mountain, stillness. Externally we have the image of wood, penetration or extension. At times, I like to ponder on this hexagram on how life proceeds unceasingly in small, sometimes imperceptible, steps and, before we know it, we are in a new place.

Returning to Australia in late 2006 after three years in China, indeed from a total of nine years of overseas comings and goings, I was so content to live in our flat by the beach in Thirroul. When not working, I enjoyed swims and walks in one of the most beautiful natural spots in the world. My taiji experience was richer for my having done it in so many beautiful places around the world, in gardens, temple grounds, parks, mountain tops, by lakes and rivers, on verandahs during torrential downpours, by the window during snow-filled mornings and more. While I had soaked in so much, to do taiji in the small park by my local beach was as inspiring as anywhere I had been around the world. And I felt the satisfaction of having done my work well, of having negotiated with so many people and situations in so many places, and with a fresh knowing that there is no end to this path of living more mindfully and letting go of the resistances in our life.

Rubing and I commuted eighty minutes each way daily to the city for work. I filled those commuting hours with a lot of catching up on books, films and music. I used this opportunity to watch the 52 part DVD series of *Romance of the Three Kingdoms*, a subtitled serialisation of one of the great epics of Chinese literature. One of the main characters is Kong Ming, also known as Zhu Ge Liang, a master tactician in war and inspiration for young readers all across Asia since the work first appeared in 1360.

One reason for reading stories about Zhu Ge Liang in the *Romance of the Three Kingdoms* is to discover new examples of the theme of achieving victory through the leverage of mind and not simply meeting force with force. Take, for example, the classic story of the empty city: One day,

Zhu Ge Liang's army finds itself low in numbers and unable to assemble enough troops to defend a particular city. The leaders were worried the people of the city would be slaughtered. But when the opposing army arrived at the entrance to the city, they met Zhu Ge Liang busy with a broom, sweeping the entrance, preparing for their welcome. He beckoned them inside. Some of the enemy leaders were eager, believing this was their big chance to take the city. Others were more cautious, thinking they were walking into a trap. Eventually the enemy army backed off and the city was saved single-handedly.

There are so many great stories about Zhu Ge Liang. One final story here is about the time he visited the south to subdue the local leader, Meng Huo, and his people. After easily being cornered, Meng Huo complained that he was just unlucky. So Zhu Ge Liang set him free and proceeded to recapture him seven times all up. When asked why he did it this way, Zhu Ge Liang stated that it was easy to physically capture him, but his goal was to capture him and his people's hearts. Here was a man committed to using mind and not force!

I found it difficult to settle back into the rhythm of working in a regional immigration office and administer what I saw as dreary government policy. I saw too much mindless action and too much force being used to apply it. Here I am particularly thinking of the computerised citizenship test which was being rushed through before the 2007 election for what I assessed to be political purposes. I hadn't sufficiently prepared myself for my return to Australia. Working in that office, I felt like I was biding my time. Waiting to again find my feet. Meanwhile, I continued to enjoy running taiji exercise classes at the local adult evening college in Wollongong.

But in the years I was away overseas, Sydney had also changed. With new generations of residents, it was as if the fringe had moved into the centre. Supermarkets were not only selling shelves and shelves of health foods, they were even stocking organic fruit and vegetables! Not so long ago, taiji and Chinese medicine were but fringe interests. Such a small percentage of the population could relate to them, let alone assess their validity in enhancing health. But by 2007, with the steady increase in Chinese migration, the situation was radically different. There was a flow of taiji teachers and practitioners of Chinese medicine from mainland China, many who claimed illustrious heritages from great teachers, coming to Australia to serve the demands of these new times. And Chinese medicine degrees had long been available in Australia.

While I continued to make taiji available locally, just as before when I was experimenting with my correspondence course in opposite meditation, I could see people's lives were getting busier than ever. I was picking up where I was before I left for overseas. While I persevered with a shortened taiji form, I knew more than ever that taiji is way more than the exercise routine many students expected. To teach the form as the form felt futile to me. I talked taiji up as a vehicle for a way of thinking, a sense of self-completeness, and as a safety valve in our faster moving life. But one can't always force these messages.

One day, while I was working in the city, I walked past the Haymarket Branch of the Sydney City Library, across the road from Sydney's original Chinatown, and there were some Chinese calligraphers offering free calligraphy for library members as part of the Chinese New Year festival. They were mostly writing characters to wish happiness and success for the new year etc, but I asked one of the old men to write: yòng yì bù yòng lì, use mind and not force, something I had been recently reading about. The experience of acquiring this piece of art, hanging in my house since that time, was a precursor to this present work.

As I witnessed the limitations of formal taiji classes to share the taiji idea, I felt driven to seek out other opportunities to express the inspiring taiji idea. I recall Simon telling me many times that it made little sense for a student to go and do the same as what their teacher had done. The great tradition of dao and taiji will always find new forms. Those who are keen can always learn the taiji form. Wanting to express myself more creatively, I decided to focus on writing, something I had only ever dabbled in over the years.

I enrolled in a creative writing course at the University of Wollongong and obtained my masters degree in prose in 2011. I revelled in this study environment. I had long wanted to write stories, but had wombled along for too many years. I did write some introductory articles about taiji in the 1980s. In the late 1980s, I even enrolled in a correspondence writing course for both fiction and nonfiction. It was a big outlay of both money and time for me to complete that course. And I succeeded in getting some short stories and articles published in magazines. It was this momentum that spurred me to develop the correspondence course in opposite philosophy and meditation which began well, but went back on the shelf when I decided to work overseas.

In my interview for admission to the writing course as a mature age student, I was asked a question of how well I had kept up with my reading. I told my interviewer that long ago I had heard some advice given by leading Australian novelist, Colleen McCullough who, when once asked what advice she would give emerging writers today, she said: 'study the classics and go out and live your life.' I told my interviewer I had obediently done both.

I never fully abandoned my writing impulses overseas as I occasionally wrote articles on taiji in the evenings. I eventually bundled these articles together and self-published them as *TAO: Total Person And One World*. This was a full expression of my passion for taiji at the time, though as mentioned at the beginning of this book often in the words of my taiji teacher. Parallel to this, I compiled a series of travel newsletters I wrote during my years overseas and self published them as *Tales of the Bear the Dragon and Other Wondrous Creatures*. While my writing began with philosophical intentions, what we may describe as geographies of the mind, they quickly became accounts of my adventures in physical locations. I didn't abandon my fiction efforts either. During my stay in Moscow I entered a short story writing contest conducted by the English language newspaper *The Moscow Times* and won second place.

After I enrolled in Creative Writing at University, I realised that after many years of working in a government department my muse took the form of a High Court judge, but now I wanted something different, that I needed to exercise a different part of my brain as I wrote.

I certainly was in a new place. During the 2009 global financial crisis, my Department offered staff the option of voluntary redundancies. Having paid off my house, and wanting to focus more on my writing, I raised my hand and gained early access to my superannuation. I left the Department with deep gratitude for the experience, for how much I had grown over nineteen years. Suddenly I found myself giving full time attention to writing. This was a fantastic opportunity. Space precludes me from going into the wonderful teachers and subjects and the inspiring environment I experienced all through my course at the

University of Wollongong. Genres I covered in my course included short and long prose, poetry, screenwriting and essay writing.

One project I must revisit is the collaborative writing project between the University of Wollongong and the University of Vigo in Spain. This project lasted four years and led to the publication by the Centre of Australian Studies in Barcelona of *The Transnational Story Hub: Between Self and Other*. The work was edited by Dr Merlinda Bobis and Dr Belen Martin-Lucas who both also conceived and guided the project. At the core of the work was study of the self and its relationship with the other. We used the discourse of transnationalism to explore this important relationship.

The project involved a series of steps, the first being our creation of sound and word images of the place where we lived and sending them to our colleagues who lived across the ocean. The next step was to exercise our imagination and creatively respond to the sound works we received. This evoked a further round of responses. Through further team discussions and workshopping, we analysed the series of exchanges to theorise about the creative process itself and our new realisations about our relationship with the other.

The result was a totally original and exciting blend of literary theory and practice (with prose, collaborative poetry and academic papers) which retained a unified focus despite the differences of approach by the dozen or so participants; the discontinuities of time, and the many fearless writing nodes willing to grow anywhere and everywhere.

In my final paper for this project, I found the best way to account for my experience was to re-engage with metaphysics and in particular phenomenology which I had studied about thirty years earlier. I had not expected this, but phenomenology re-emerged from the depths of my awareness.

Along the way, in seeking to understand the contemporary theories in the self and other, I could find no clearer image of the interaction of self and other than in the taiji exercise of Pushing Hands mentioned in an earlier chapter. This physical exercise bridges the distances we set up between ourselves through language. In this exercise, we shape our own movement as others shape theirs. We help ourselves to be better able to help others, and we seek improvement in others so that we can find more improvement in ourselves. Yin and yang are never separated. This is our mental comprehension because of how they are written as two separate words on the page, but yin endlessly supports yang just as yang supports yin. This is the taiji symbol, the concept of yin and yang always working together. But Pushing Hands is a metaphor for our relationship with the other and we do not need to be physically present to gain the benefit of the spirit of this exercise.

In my fictional writing projects since university, perhaps even before that, I have been guided by an idea that, as humans, we will live a better life when we have some sort of metaphysical framework which allows for our growth in the understanding of the nonphysical world. As I embarked on writing novels, I can see, in hindsight, that I created characters whose flaws could be traced back to various metaphysical misconceptions. I explored situations where people dealt with such failings to find their way forward in life. I guess that period of writing has stimulated me to write more directly about metaphysics as I understand it and hence this book.

As a hobby, over years, not imagining I would pen such a full length book as this, I have enjoyed writing poetry to capture moments of my experience with taiji and martial art world in general, and in 2016, I realised that I had enough poems to form a collection so I published it as *Pick Up the Pearl*.

23 Extending taiji

One who takes up taiji, who becomes familiar with the idea behind the taiji form, and who even vaguely knows what they like, will effortlessly find themselves applying the taiji idea in their own life in new and often unique ways. This book is a reflection of how I have taken my taiji along a philosophical path so that now I can share the fruits of this journey with others in this way. I have taiji friends who are highly unlikely to ever pick up a philosophy book. But they are very good at what they do, whether it be in the teaching, healing or other professions. Many people over the centuries have applied taiji to their own interests and while martial arts throws up some eye-catching case studies, it is is but one such application.

A taiji teacher will teach taiji knowing their students will take it to a new place. We don't need to encourage people to extend their taiji because it is a natural and spontaneous process that cannot be stopped. After committing to a few core principles, there is no standardising taiji. I always revel in seeing fresh examples of how the taiji idea is extended into new fields of activity. It's as if I feel a close affinity with people I may never meet in person.

This precedent goes back a long way. In Chinese philosophy, the word dao is used as a description of the way of the universe. But there is also the meaning of a way a person does things. Of course, the person who is aligned with the macrocosmic dao will demonstrate that dao in their own microcosmic world. Daoist philosopher, Zhuang Zi, often extolled a philosophy of nature in his writings with much humour. He tells stories of characters who had their own dao-based way of doing things. For example, he writes about the man who could enter the wild water rapids and flow with the water and resurface without getting hurt because he followed the dao of the water. Elsewhere he comments that even thieves have their own dao. And he tells the famous story of Cook Ting who knew how to wield a knife so that it never went blunt:

> Cook Ting was cutting up an ox for Lord Wen-hui. As every touch of his hand, every heave of his shoulder, every move of his feet, every thrust of his knee — zip!

zoop! He slithered the knife along with a zing, and all was in perfect rhythm, as though he were performing the dance of the Mulberry Grove or keeping time to the Ching-shou music.

"Ah, this is marvelous!" said Lord Wen-hui. "Imagine skill reaching such heights!"

Cook Ting laid down his knife and replied, "What I care about is the Way, which goes beyond skill. When I first began cutting up oxen, all I could see was the ox itself. After three years I no longer saw the whole ox. And now — now I go at it by spirit and don't look with my eyes. Perception and understanding have come to a stop and spirit moves where it wants. I go along with the natural makeup, strike in the big hollows, guide the knife through the big openings, and following things as they are. So I never touch the smallest ligament or tendon, much less a main joint.

"A good cook changes his knife once a year — because he cuts. A mediocre cook changes his knife once a month — because he hacks. I've had this knife of mine for nineteen years and I've cut up thousands of oxen with it, and yet the blade is as good as though it had just come from the grindstone. There are spaces between the joints, and the blade of the knife has really no thickness. If you insert what has no thickness into such spaces, then there's plenty of room — more than enough for the blade to play about it. That's why after nineteen years the blade of my knife is still as good as when it first came from the grindstone.

"However, whenever I come to a complicated place, I size up the difficulties, tell myself to watch out and be careful, keep my eyes on what I'm doing, work very slowly, and move the knife with the greatest subtlety, until — flop! the whole thing comes apart like a clod of earth crumbling to the ground. I stand there holding the knife and look all around me, completely satisfied and reluctant to move on, and then I wipe off the knife and put it away."

"Excellent!" said Lord Wen-hui. "I have heard the words of Cook Ting and learned how to care for life!" (translated by Burton Watson, 1964)

At this point I want to introduce two useful examples which are much closer to home.

Swimming

Total Immersion (TI) is a style of swimming founded by Terry Laughlin (1951-2017) which resonates deeply with the principles of taiji. It's a type of swimming yoga. Taught through a series of drills which break down each element of the swimming stroke, the swimmer consciously relaxes and monitors themselves for good form, seeking to feel the buoyancy, the streamlining sensation, the non-resistance and the flow through the water as their first points of focus. They leave strength and distance as inevitable outcomes which come in their own time. Laughlin says: 'Here, fitness is something that happens to you while you practice good technique.'

Terry Laughlin was a big fan of open water swimming. He talked about his participation in swims around Manhattan Island, a length of 28 kilometres, claiming that he would be almost as fresh at the end of that swim as he was at the beginning because of the way he swam.

Swimming as taught in the past was often little more than organised struggle as we essentially learned how not to drown. Sometimes I ask people what having a good swim feels like, and sadly some think it means pain or feeling spent after meeting a pre-set goal. Despite the prevalence of miseducation in swimming technique, young champions regularly arrive on the scene to swim a more natural style and Terry Laughlin concluded these were the ones to show the best way forward. He made a close study of natural champions and sought to catalogue the elements of their styles which could be taught. For example, over and over again, he noticed champions used less strokes per length of the pool, something which sounds wrong to those who believe in the brawn-based approach to fast swimming. Velocity equals the product of stroke length and stroke rate and it turns out that stroke length, achieved through skill, let's say brain-based, has a more significant impact on speed than stroke rate.

Even when we take a step forward and attend to a swimmer's psychological condition to improve their performance, we may be only mounting up the force and the consequent resistance if we do not find a better physical technique that does not rely on fighting with the water.

A key element in Total Immersion swimming is to reduce the resistance against the water. The more horizontal we are in the water the less drag we will experience. The lower half of the body of many beginners drags through the water. However when we realise that the lungs are a cushion of air, when we press our chests into the water, our hips will rise and the lower half of our body will automatically lift and align more horizontally with the surface of the water. We feel like we are swimming downhill.

With Total Immersion, we train ourselves to never enter the struggle zone. To illustrate my point about our misconceptions of the virtue of struggle, I refer to the example of Russian swimmer, Alexander Popov, one of the greatest sprint swimmers of all time and who won gold in the 50 metres and 100 metres sprint in two Olympic Games in a row. Laughlin points out how Popov practised good swimming stroke habits many hours per day and he often swam relatively slow laps to build these habits. Onlookers seriously doubted his ability to win big sprint races because was wasn't working out hard and pushing himself to the limit. However, Popov's focus was to build the muscle memory, and improve each element of his stroke so that when the moment came to compete, his body would perform.

I practise Total Immersion skills in my regular swims at my local pool, and it is a total pleasure to be able to apply my taiji idea in this form. I resonate with the drills because of my taiji and my morning taiji is richer for my swimming practice.

Chirunning

Danny and Katherine Dreyer have written about ChiRunning, a form of running which they describe as a revolutionary approach to effortless, injury-free running. In summary, it is about learning a good posture for our body, so that our body can best operate as a whole while we are running. One important key is that we keep our body in a straight line and we lean forward from the ankles, so that our foot strikes the ground behind the body's centre of gravity leading to less impact on the body, much less resistance than if we lagged behind the strike. In this way, running becomes an exercise in controlled falling. It is about letting gravity do all the work and us not resisting it.

Again, it's all about resistance. When we watch children running around in play we see them balanced and centred often while they have smiles on their faces. There is a theory that running is as much a part of our evolutionary make-up as is walking. The theory goes that our biology reflects a natural affinity for running. The Dreyers claim that it is not running that ever causes injuries to people, but the form of the running. We have lost a lot of the natural impulses and instead run with so many habits of resistance.

Danny Dreyer was already a long distance runner when he became more interested in meditation and even taiji exercise itself. When he went to live in San Francisco, he met a taiji master in the local park, a person named George Xu, and told he told Master Xu that he wanted to learn taiji from him to incorporate taiji principles into his running, not just to do taiji for its own sake. George Xu agreed to help.

ChiRunning is about getting our body to work as a whole where all the parts are working for each other, not against each other. We will know when we haven't got that right, because we will feel pain. So even injuries are working for us because they are pointing out parts of our form that need to be improved. I know this from personal experience as I have learned from my heels, my ankles, shins, and knees how to improve my posture.

As in taiji, the strength of the runner comes from the full length of the spine and the limbs need to be relaxed to become extensions of that strength emanating from the spine. So the five key principles of ChiRunning as presented by the Dreyers are much the same as taiji exercise principles:
1. Cotton and Steel - we find our strength in the centre of our body, and outwardly we are relaxed and flexible;
2. Gradual Progress – we move towards our big goal in a series of small steps;
3. The Pyramid – the smaller system is supported by the larger system;

4. Balance in Motion – again, quietness in movement and movement in quietness;
5. Nonidentification – with good posture and form we can train our mind to be like an ideal government, no longer holding us back but encouraging us forwards.

Again, like Total Immersion swimming, ChiRunning is not about speed or distance. The principles and drills can be practised on small runs. Our running routine will grow naturally without any need for forced routines. I used to love running when I was at school, it was part of our training for our football. I stopped for many years, Actually coming back from China one day I decided to go to the local oval and have a run, I quickly developed shin splints. I talked to a few medics who told me to give running away because I would never get over them. It was about this time, I came across the Dreyer's book and I have enjoyed many runs on bush trails, in parks and along the road in the years since. It is again for me, a way to revel in more taiji application.

24 Attitude

'When you ask: 'Who am I?' you are trying to read yourself as if you were a simple sentence already written. Instead, you write yourself as you go along. The sentence that you recognise is only one of many probable variations. You and no other choose which experiences you want to actualise. ' Seth in *The Nature of the Psyche*

As I was penning my first draft of this book, I felt the urge to avoid descension into didactic detail about taiji as it is taught in so many schools and discussed on so many online groups, and from that I gave birth to the desire to render the art of taiji into the most creative, colourful and complete form words could convey which, as per its Daoist heritage, I have previously defined as the taiji of no taiji (a la 'the taiji that can be told is not the true taiji') and that meant divesting its physical form of its postures, the usual method of transmission of taiji thought and, as a consequence, the book of associated photographs of each posture with their barely translatable names, and it meant moving to a more general place, to the broader concept, as per the philosophy books, think yin yang symbol, and how the taiji concept can become a source of such insight into dealing with daily life, the operative idea being yin for yang and yang for yin, a subject that can always be beneficially expanded upon, and it was at this time that I settled upon the keyword 'attitude' to best express where I was coming from and where we could go with taiji without having learned and practised its individual postures, postures as various as 'crossing hands to catch the seven stars' or 'take the tiger by the legs and punch him in the belly', but, to my surprise, when I sought out the dictionary definition of the word 'attitude', I discovered that it very much means posture, like the posture of a sculpture, a settled mode of thinking, more specifically, the etymological source defines attitude as 'a posture in the body supposed to imply a mental state', so that if we now fast forward to today, the word has been reborn as something different, having become disembodied, let's say an out-of-body posture, though thankfully it's a word we all know well without too much argument, and so it is still capable of serving my current purposes, perhaps even adding new dimensions to our taiji understanding, akin to a performance of eurhythmy, developed as a whole new language of body movement that unites inner and outer worlds, and which may be worthy of attention some other time but for now I return my focus onto our chosen word having made the short shift from the physical posture to the mental one, which, to repeat, at least enables me to communicate the intended idea via the written word without the need for a physical demonstration, and here is a good place to remind my reader that, in my use of the written word to express my thoughts on the importance of attitude, I am also seizing the opportunity to use the writing itself (theorists call it extradiegetic) to be yet another example of the attitude I am seeking to describe, that is, the written form of this chapter, with its widely cast, let me call them dragnet sentences, which gather so many fleeting, tenuously related thoughts which refuse to conform to the usual neatly packaged sentence format, but they work together and influence each other, in their many associations, references and impressions, to create a more honest picture about the complexity of the human condition, and which allows me to reinforce the theme of taiji as being about the greater whole, while its various parts remain flexible, continuous and well-connected, with commas serving as joints, allowing us to pause momentarily to catch our breath, while never cutting off the flow entirely, and yet lending flexibility, reach and co-ordination as we investigate the whys and hows of the taiji attitude, which are actually based on sound scientific principles as I am about to argue, so we are all clear that we don't profess attitude for attitude's sake alone, but rather for the sake of that greater whole which resonates with and merges with the totality of all that we are.

Those wary souls who yawn at another's seemingly rabid insistence to find a more positive attitude to life, those souls who kindly look away when others bang on too much about how a better attitude will do us all the world of good, those who are numbed at the repeated bidding of others who claim that success is all about attitude full stop, flogging and re-flogging that dead horse, they are all correct in their disinclination to listen, in that it get's so tiring to hear such admonitions out of context, they hear words that disappear into thin air, for they have no gravitas, no energy and no feeling, the listener sees fingers pointing to nowhere of any interest to them, but, oh, once we do see the context, in this case, the scientific basis for why attitude matters, ahead lies an endless path of discovery lined with joy after joy as we realise just how we are part of that greater being which is creative by its very nature, and the argument is very simply put: namely that we, at our core are made of a nonphysical creative substance, and as we engage with our ever expanding world, we replicate that world, and there is a method to this replication, much in the same way that the Buddhists claim that the focus of our attention is the most precious of our possessions because whatever we focus our attention upon is what grows in our experience, prompting us to ask that simple question of whether, right now, we are focusing on what we want or on what we don't want, as the creative substance which lies at our neutral core delivers more of what ever it is we are staring at, as if it has studied absolute mathematics seeing the absolute value of both positive one and negative one as simply one, it continues to replicate our version of events and we always have choices about that, and this is echoed in other teachings of the ages, for example in the works of Plato, a great advocate of the achievement of freedom through knowledge, and yet a person who strongly believed in censorship as part of any education system because he believed that the creative substance which young people are learning to wield will simply re-create whatever it is that is shown to them and so it made good sense to fill their senses with examples of beauty, harmony and divine order for that is what they will, in turn, re-create in their own experience, and so we can begin to see how a person who remains focused on the positive aspects of their experience will attract more positive experiences and a person who harps on negative moments will attract more negative moments, and of course we can all find examples in our own lives of people who attract such fortune or misfortune.

The theme of this book, its main idea or what, if the book was an entity in its own right, we could call the 'me' of this book is the use of mind and not force, a phrase borrowed from Yang Cheng Fu's written legacy to the taiji tradition, and used in particular reference to the execution of a taiji move, but also a phrase which we can use to guide us to achieve our goals in life more generally, though we do need to clarify that, when we break this phrase down into the dichotomy of thought and action, we are not dismissing action, nor are we advocating thought at the expense of action, as if mind power alone will help us achieve all of our goals, or even simply mindfulness, but rather we do see thought and action as being on two opposite sides of the same circle, reinforcing, feeding and balancing each other, so that there is a place for action, but it is preferable that this action be balanced by clear thinking, which is not a revolutionary idea, not new for sure, as it is a principle we follow much of the time in all of our personal and social activities, for example think about the construction of buildings, where we don't rush in straight away and build, build, build, do, do, do but rather find the right people with the right understanding to draw up the plans and have those plans checked, so that the location, the foundations, the materials, the design and all the rest are appropriate for the desired building, a good example to consider how we are already familiar with this interplay of thought and action in the course of our everyday lives, but sometimes we do forget and we fall under the illusion of action as being the solution to whatever problem we encounter, and are repeatedly reminded that the problem with inappropriate action is that too often we meet resistance that can leave us short of our goal and also feeling very tired, whereas a better understanding of the relationship between thought and action can lead us into a state of actionless action where, of course, we exert force in our life activities, but it is with the minimum force required and this can become so easy it almost feels like the force of no force at all.

I digress here to demonstrate an important point in this chapter with an example which, though it is very close to home, does need some introductory background as it is to do with my previously mentioned poetry book, *Pick Up The Pearl,* the title of which comes from another taiji posture, 'pick up the pearl from the bottom of the ocean and lift it to the top of the boat', a book of poetry about the experience of learning and practising taiji and also about taiji-related subjects such as wushu and martial arts, as well as the Yi Jing, which underpins much of the theory of taiji, in fact, the Yi Jing contains one of the first written references to the word taiji itself, so, in summary, the poems were all related to my personal taiji journey and I thought they would be worth sharing with people on a similar journey and so I offered them to a taiji facebook group of several thousand people, and I was surprised to receive a reply from the group administrator that it wasn't appropriate to upload the collection, and accompanying the reason given was that too many people try to add random martial arts items to the group and it was his duty to delete all posts not directly related to taiji when he sees them, and he added that he had to be vigilant and set boundaries, I suppose to protect what he believed to be taiji, though I was left wondering how can this person and members of his group deepen their experience of taiji, when the administrator has pre-judged what taiji is, and he has actually set boundaries to refuse whatever he considers to not be taiji, especially when we know that the original meaning of the word taiji is often translated as that thing without limit, all adding up to a very puzzling experience, though I have to admit an experience which offered me rich insight into people's attitudes in general when they start setting conditions in all the different areas of life, and even taiji masters today do it, whereas at least in this case, the study of taiji is really the study of the unconditional nature of our nonphysical being, and yet we impose our finite understanding as if it is absolute, and wonder again why we meet both resistance and more and more unwanted conditions, leading to a society so confused about so many things in life, and so bewildered with our inability to control and set conditions, and sadly even indignant when we can't see the beginning or the end of our eternal experience.

Taiji is the word we have agreed to use in this book to encapsulate the idea of using mind and not force, but we are actually dealing with a perennial idea, an idea abundantly expressed in numerous ways across our culture, and in fact across all cultures whatever their time or place, and it is endlessly rewarding to toy with fresh examples, fresh utterances of this idea, as if to reinforce our understanding of the benefit of this knowledge and to inspire us to find resonance with who we really are so that we too may express it in our own unique way, leaving us with a seeming wealth of precious gems laying at our feet in a way that whenever we feel the inclination we can pick any one of those gems up and give it a polish, and marvel in the light it throws, and here I am prompted to flag one such example laid at our feet hundreds of years ago to illustrate how even as children we clearly understand the value of using mind over sheer physical force, so here I wish to recount in summary form one of Grimm's fairy tales, which fell into my field of vision even as I was writing this chapter, and this is the story of *The Valiant Little Tailor:*

Upright in his chair by the front window of his house, a rather optimistic young man, whom we shall call the valiant little tailor, though he is also known in some versions of the story as Master Snip, was in high spirits and sewing away, when a lady selling jam walked past in the street and the valiant little tailor sweet-talked her into giving him four ounces of jam, for which he was very grateful and this led him to pray that something good would come from this jam, which it did in the form of seven flies which landed on that jam and couldn't be shooed away driving the valiant little tailor to swat them after which he felt so proud about his new found valour that he immediately embroidered the message onto his belt: 'seven in one blow', and as he thought about his brave act, he decided his sewing table was too small for a man such as himself and so he decided to head out to see the world, putting in his pocket before he left one piece of cheese from the kitchen and a bird he found caught in a thicket outside his house, in even higher spirits than when he woke up, and dearly hoping the world could read those words on his belt: 'seven in one blow' which is what, in fact, a giant walking along the same road did and that giant quickly came to the conclusion that the words meant that this little man had killed seven people with one blow and so he had better be careful in talking with him, and the story continues with the valiant little tailor hoodwinking the giant, in the first test of strength by squeezing the chunk of cheese as if it was a stone, and in the second test by throwing the bird in the air, and as it flew away the giant thought the tailor had thrown a stone further than he could see, so that once he had gained the confidence of this first giant he next tricked that giant and his giant friend into a fight where they both killed each other, and with his indomitable attitude, the valiant little tailor went on, after a few more displays of skill based on his clever use of mind, married the king's daughter and gained half of the kingdom, a lovely demonstration of how less can be more expressed in a way that even children can understand.

Delving further in the nature of attitude, it is opportune for us to once again don our phenomenology hat, our strategy of seeing the things themselves and letting them speak from their essence, and consider attitude as being that posture of the mind, let's remember it's a dynamic posture, ever changing, not a posture fixed once and for all, and while we know we can't apply physical laws to the realm of the nonphysical, we do know that the nonphysical does seek expression into the physical world, so we can observe the effects of attitude, though we can't define it, and its at this point I share the words of Lao Zi where he describes the people aligned with nature as follows:

The ancient masters were subtle, mysterious, profound, responsive, the depth of their knowledge is unfathomable, because it is unfathomable, all we can do is describe their appearance, watchful, like men crossing a winter stream, alert, like men aware of danger, courteous, like visiting guests, yielding, like ice about to melt, simple, like uncarved blocks of wood, hollow, like caves, opaque, like muddy pools, who can wait quietly while the mud settles? who can remain still until the moment of action? Observers of the Tao do not seek fulfillment, not seeking fulfillment, they are not swayed by desire for change (DDC Chapter 15).

Eventually, everybody gets the idea, so why not today?

25 Immortality

When I began taiji classes, my most immediate desired outcome, as it was for most beginners, was to get healthier. The stretching and relaxing action of the muscles of both our limbs and core body, as well as the subtle massage effect on our internal organs, made a lot of sense. This was before we learned about the activation of the qi meridians to assist energy flow through our body as a way to increased vitality.

Very early on, I obtained a copy of the previously discussed Zhang San Feng's treatise on taiji where in the endnote he stated that he wanted people of the world to attain longevity and not just martial art skills. This conventional take on taiji appealed to me.

However, by the time I was researching taiji for my honours thesis, I discovered a central theme of Daoism, so entwined with the taiji tradition, is immortality, and the history of Daoism was loaded with stories about the quest for immortality. It employs an almost endless number of symbols and phrases about this subject. We most popularly have the peach of immortality that is grown in heaven, and we have those Daoists who, at an agreed time, assume the form of a white crane and fly off across to the ocean of immortality. The suggestion was always physical immortality. The line between life extension and immortality appears very blurred.

All through Chinese history, we can read about semi-mythical characters who lived in remote places, people who often fed only on the air and who seemed to merge with the environment at will, manifesting to mortals and then disappearing again over long periods of time. When so eloquently portrayed in literature, they certainly stir the imagination. Some accounts of Zhang San Feng portray him as one such character.

In Chinese history, the traditional methods to achieve immortality can be divided into two types: a) religious: meditation, rituals etc; or b) physical: diets, medicines, breathing techniques, exercises and good deeds. The Chinese folk tradition has a huge lore of remedies, from plants, animals and the earth, that can deal with almost any human situation including mortality. This has given birth to the Chinese herbal and pharmacological medicine as we know it today. It is inevitable there would be numerous attempts to create the pill of immortality, And of course there always seemed to be buyers.

As a citizen of the twenty-first century, I do desire to live a long and happy life. While I have never felt the urge to seek the elixir of immortality, I have long been fascinated by this tradition and always wanted to know what these stories were all about.

In the Western tradition, there are also legends similar to the more outlandish stories of the Daoist tradition. One such example is Count de St Germain, often described as an emissary of a mystery school. We have accounts of people meeting him as a fit and healthy middle-aged man, from the early 1700s to the mid-1800s. He was recognised as an outstanding scholar and linguist and was a widely travelled diplomat known and respected by many crowned heads of European states and beyond. He had a close association with secret occult societies and claimed a whole range of unusual skills such as the ability to remove flaws from jewellery, and of course he was able to prepare an elixir of immortality. There are still groups of people around the world today who claim to be in communication with this person at the vibrational level. Again, wearing the hat of the phenomenologist, I have always wanted to know what the people who study this subject were getting at.

I have already described how my early schooling was closely integrated with church life. Our primary school was located next to our church, besides which was the school auditorium and the presbytery for the several priests who lived in the town. From about seven years old to fourteen, I served as an altar boy at this church. I was on a roster which meant that for one week about every month, I would have to get out of bed early and do the twenty minute walk to church to serve for the 7am mass, before returning home for breakfast and heading back to school for a 9am start. It was okay in the summer months but it made winters seem very long and cold.

One of the duties of the altar boys was to assist the priest at funeral services. On the occasion of a death of a parishioner, a mass was held at the church before the mourners moved on to the cemetery for the burial rites as the coffin was lowered into the ground. By the age of fourteen I had attended many funerals. One stand out memory from these events was the phrase: 'may eternal life be granted unto him (or her)'. 'Eternal life' is a phrase often used in the Catholic liturgy and which I will explore further below, but it did seem paradoxical to me that people gathered to pray for eternal life for a person who had just supposedly died. Call it my homespun anthropology if you like, but I came to the early conclusion that whatever form an afterlife took, funerals were conducted primarily to console the people who remained.

It is curious that our Catholic education contained little explanation of the afterlife beyond the existence of a place called heaven where nothing ever seemed to happen. I accept that the Catholic church prefers to teach with simplistic images and concepts. This is an important plank in any good communication strategy. But the widespread view today is that the concept of heaven is a tool used by the powerful to cow and blackmail others to do what is asked of them. So heaven has become a tarnished concept for so many in the modern world and with that there is little thought of an afterlife.

The Apostle's Creed which is said during the Catholic Mass contains the lines: 'I believe in the resurrection of the body and life everlasting'. The New Testament has many occurrences of the same phrase, for example when St Paul writes to the Romans in The Epistles, he says: 'the wages of sin is death; but the free gift of God is eternal life in Christ Jesus Our Lord.'

One of the most well known parables of Jesus Christ is that of the Good Samaritan. This story is introduced when a lawyer asks Christ:

'What must I do to inherit eternal life?'

Jesus asks him, 'What is written in the law? How do you read it?'

The lawyer replies: 'You shall love the lord your God with all your heart, with all your soul, with all your strength, with all your mind, and your neighbour as yourself.'

Jesus tells him: 'You have answered correctly. Do this and you will live.'

But the lawyer continues with the question: 'And who is my neighbour?'

From here Jesus launches into the parable of the Good Samaritan.

So we were strongly encouraged to care for other people for many reasons, but exactly what 'eternal life' is, was never explained to us. And I don't remember anybody questioning the concept at the time. Of course, much of religion is a matter of faith, which means beyond question. More often than not, anyone who is uncertain will put that issue on hold and think about more pressing issues in life.

I have no doubt that there is benefit in talking of immortality and eternal life. I do not agree with the sceptics who dismiss it all as a meaningless waste of time.

Firstly, I see such talk as being an expression of an intuitive understanding that some part of us remains un-incarnated in our earthly experience, and that part of us is what we may describe as eternal. As human beings engaged in our myriad daily activities, it is easy for us to forget this connection. And there is much that flows from this forgetting. We begin to form false assumptions about life and the world around us and these can be detrimental to our well-being. It can be a play of remembering and forgetting, and such play is often fun. For example, after we forget where we put our keys, we feel so happy when we find them. It is this human forgetfulness that inspires teachers and artists to create works that will remind us in new and engaging ways something so fundamental to our being.

There is the question of whether this connection with the eternal is a fact or is a belief. But again science is validating a lot of traditional knowledge. In cell theory, there is a clear law that all cells come from cells (Latin: omnis cellula e cellula). And each of these cells carry complex genetic codes which are shared across species. Life has never ceased to be in the whole history of the universe. It is immortal. So the question is whether we are part of that or not. But even if it is merely belief, the question becomes can this belief help us to live a happier life?

Here I would like to relate a conversation between renowned Daoism author, John Blofeld, and a recluse who went by the name of Moon

Rabbit Recluse and who lived in a Daoist community on Hua Shan Mountain, not far from the city of Xi'An. The recluse said:

> 'Immortals not only break wind or belch like other people, they die! Can it ever have been otherwise? Becoming immortal has little to do with physical changes, like the greying of a once glossy black beard; it means coming to know something, realising something – an experience that can happen in a flash! Ah, how precious is that knowledge! When it first strikes you, you want to sing and dance, or you nearly die of laughing! For suddenly you recognise that nothing in the world can ever hurt you. Though thunder roars and torrents boil, though serpents hiss and arrows rain – you meet them with laughter! You see your body as a flower born to bloom, to give forth fragrance, to wither and to die. Who would care for a peony as it was for a lifetime, for a thousand or ten thousand years? A mere cabbage would be worthier of attention. It is well that things die when they are worn out, and no loss at all, for life is immortal and never grows with the birth of things or diminishes with their death. A worn out object is discarded, life having ample materials to supply the loss. Now do you see? You cannot die because you have never lived. Life cannot die, because it has no beginning or end. Becoming an immortal just means ceasing to identify yourself with shadows and recognising that the only 'you' is everlasting life. Ah, what nonsense I am talking.'

This is where I bring it around to my morning practise of taiji and how this exercise is a beautiful model of a process, with its many circular postures, that has no beginning and no end. Focusing on this exercise and its many related images can be soothing to the mind as I am immersed within a world of seeming interruption and discontinuity. We survived changes of seasons, residence, employment, circles of friends, interests and life projects, and amongst all of those changes, we can still feel a sense of continuity.

And using taiji as a meditation on our total being, we learn to feel our connection to that un-incarnated part of us, which has never know imbalance, suffering, lack or whatever. And it is refreshing and energising to invest a small amount of time each day in this activity of blending with that un-incarnated part of my self..

Even though I have studied taiji and related Daoist philosophy for forty years, if someone were to ask me what is my religion or philosophy, I wouldn't call myself a Daoist. I have the religion of no religion, the same as the first Daoists, or even the first Christians before they were called so. I usually reply that I simply believe in nature. There is no better word to capture my perspective. I find that God is a word that, while it has worked well in past for the purposes of transmission of religious teaching, it has been misused too often. The original meaning is lost. As Nietzsche proclaimed: *God is dead*. I know exactly what he was getting at. Of course, the real God is not dead and is as eternal as ever. But we are all numb from the religious God we have had forced upon us for too long. The real and eternal God is right here all about us, has never deserted us, and is never making adverse judgments on me or any other person. Those of mainstream religion have a different understanding. I fully accept that the world is teeming with godliness, but I do not wish to add to the ignorance that has become our present world's 'God' teaching.

I look forward to new and more colourful ways that people communicate the eternal nature of being and our enjoyable and dramatic participation in this game. And I see that we are moving closer to the wonderful realisation that we are the creators of our own reality in more ways than we presently imagine. Of course, we share many perimeters on our beliefs that we need to go along with, but those new stories will nourish us in ways we can question our present day limitations helping us to let go of that trail of resistance we have collected along the eternal way.

26 Alchemy

'Curious enquirer into All That Is
Whose guiding principle and end I sought,
The hidden gold I spied within th' abyss,
Made it my leaven, to fulfilment brought.
Then I explained how in a mother's womb
The soul makes house, and how the pip and crumb
Of vine and corn, sealed in their earthy tomb
By miracle the bread and wine become.
The void; God spoke; the void became a thing;
I doubted this — for what maintained it so?
Nought but the void was ground and scaffolding.
At last, with scales that blame and merit show,
I weighed the eternal and it called to me;
I died adoring it, no more I know.'
(Comte de Saint-Germain trans by Sebastian Hayes)

Having sought, in the last chapter, to locate immortality as part of my complete taiji understanding, I now continue with an account of the practice of alchemy. These two noble pursuits are often bundled together as if they are the same thing. I guess sometimes there is value in teachers being a little hazy and not wishing to define their terms too clearly: it gives students more scope for their own discovery.

A key skill we learn in performing our taiji postures is to harmonise opposing physical forces. We don't achieve this by manipulating either of those forces but rather by putting ourselves into the centre of the motion where we see each force as part of a single flow. From that centre we can better direct those forces without any need to resist them. For example, from the centre, we see how the two seeming antagonistic forces of motion up and motion down are in fact part of the same circle. Motion forwards and backwards, left and right tell a similar story. We train ourselves to see through the eyes of the centre of the motion.

A major outcome of meditation is a harmony of opposites. This type of meditation goes by many names and some people call it inner alchemy. Those who master inner alchemy often claim special strength and powers, one of the greatest of which is to heal disease.

Inner alchemy of course suggests an outer alchemy. In its simplest form, the outer, or let's say physical, process of alchemy is historically linked to the tradition of turning lead and other base metals into gold.

Perhaps as an individual, I am impressionable by nature. Or it could be that I am one of an impressionable generation. But when people talk and write about this form of alchemy my imagination becomes fired up. The thought of all this gold sparks my mind as I imagine the possibilities. And I am not alone in this fascination with gold. We all know about the waves of gold fever that have swept the world in earlier times. People of all stations in life would stop what they were doing, walk away from their travails and, with the barest of essentials, hurry off to the site of the latest gold strike. Think of California in the 1840s, Australia in the 1850s and Alaska in the 1890s to name a few examples.

Regarding the seemingly implausible process of physical alchemy, remember that I had a Catholic education where I was raised to believe in miracles. We were schooled daily on the many stories of Jesus performing his miracles as well as others who acted in his name. However, as we shall learn, the Church very much claims a monopoly on miracles, either ridiculing or administering much worse treatment to those who seek to achieve miracles in their own workshops.

In teaching taiji, Simon never used the word 'alchemy' but he was firmly fixed on the original idea of harmonising yin and yang forces as a means to developing inner strength and its ensuing healing, teaching and harmonising powers. The Chinese character for healing is an ideogram of a person using a bow to shoot an arrow at a target. For people like Simon, the word 'miracle' made little sense. People simply do what they do and become good at it. Here I am reminded of that comment from Wolfgang Mozart: 'Don't ask me how I write music. I write music in the same way cows piss.'

There is a case to be made that once we begin to use the word 'alchemy' many are already turned off from what we are saying. But over the years

I have followed my whim and explored the subject as it has been documented by so many writers.

The history of alchemy is a rich subject for the phenomenologist. While it has a poetry and a promise that resonates deeply within the human soul, here is a phenomenon that is loaded with a series of unexamined presuppositions, a bevy of myths and lore, a string of inflated expectations and a litany of hundredth hand accounts accumulated over many centuries, all which can easily leave a newcomer to the subject asking a lot of hard questions.

The Chinese tradition of alchemy has been aligned with inner alchemy and immortality for a far longer time than the Western tradition. When Chinese alchemists produced gold, they freely acknowledged they were producing synthetic or fake gold as the main purpose in producing it was to ingest it to give the human body special powers, particularly longevity.

There are many stories associated with these alchemical activities over the centuries. Consider the story of Cheng Wei. She achieved the elixir but then got beaten by her husband who wanted it for himself. In response to the beating, she killed herself. And she was so close to immortality!

The *Cantong Qi* (*The Kinship of the Three*) one of the earliest overt Chinese alchemical texts, reputed to have been written by alchemist Wei Boyang in the second century AD, focuses very much on the inner processes of alchemy and seems to suggest a rare simplicity about the process. Alchemy in this tradition was not about making gold to get rich quick. In an early section of the *Cantong Qi*, Wei comments:

> The arts are so many- for each thousand, there are ten thousand more.
> Their tortuous routes run against the Yellow Emperor and the Old Master,
> their winding courses oppose Nine Capitals.
> Those who are bright comprehend the meaning of this:
> in all its breadth they know where it comes from.
> (trans Fabrizio Pregadio)

Though its destination is perhaps the same, Western alchemy has certainly travelled a different path. In that alchemy's root word, *al-kīmiya* from Arabic actually means 'the Egyptian science', there is speculation that the phenomenon may go back thousands of years to the Egyptian Empire.

In the Western tradition, there is an enduring narrative about the particular art of turning lead into gold. Manly Palmer Hall, an occult researcher and teacher claimed that over one hundred thousand manuscripts existed on the subject before the printing press was introduced in the mid-1400s.

Hall also lists some of the most well known names associated with this pursuit: Thomas Norton, Isaac of Holland, Basil Valentine, Jean de Meung, Roger Bacon, Albertus Magnus, Quercentanus Gerber, Paracelsus, Nicholas Flamel, John Frederick Helvetius, Raymond Lully, Alexander Sethon, Michael Sendivogius, Count Bernard of Trevigo, Sir George Ripley, Picus de Mirandola, John Dee, Henry Kunrath, Michael Maier, Thomas Vaughan, J B von Helmont, John Heydon, Lascaris, Thomas Charmock, Synesius, Morieu, Compte di Cagliostro, and Comte de St-Germain.

On 13 January 1404, Henry IV (1367-1413) of England passed a law that declared the multiplying of metals to be a crime against the crown. His concern was that a rush of gold into the monetary supply would damage the economy. This law, in part, read: 'None from henceforth should use to multiply Gold or Silver or use the craft of multiplication, and if any the same do they shall incur the pain of penalty.'

When William of Orange and Mary II ascended the throne of England in 1689, they repealed the above law. Robert Boyle and Isaac Newton were two of those who lobbied strongly for this repeal. The decision given was that the law had driven those who exercise the art into foreign territories and this was clearly to the detriment of the economy of the local realm.

Still today, records buried in libraries and private collections around the world contain eyewitness accounts of the transformation of lead, silver, tin and other metals into gold. How do we deal with such phenomena? When I see the misrepresentation of life in our present day even as it is being recorded, I have always questioned how well we can even know what people were really doing, let alone thinking, in times long ago.

We do know, however, that in medieval times, each of the different known metals were seen as being located on a hierarchy with lead being the lowest and gold being the highest. This was way before the periodic table was ever formulated. The mindset of the alchemist was to raise the purity of lead to that of gold through a range of what we would call chemical processes. The most dedicated alchemists emphasised that there needed to be a corresponding purification of the practitioner for the process to work correctly.

About the form of physical alchemy, in that it is associated with so many cultures and traditions over thousands of years, at the very minimum we must accept as a steppingstone on the path of human knowledge from which many benefits have come. Alchemy played a valuable role as a precursor to the science of chemistry in the way it stimulated researchers to ask many fundamental questions about the physical world and this lead to some very beneficial answers. I see that ultimately our opinion on this subject comes down to belief, and as we are free creative agents who can choose to believe what ever we wish. And depending on what we do believe, we will attract evidence supporting that belief and we will dismiss conflicting evidence. With this in mind, I claim that physical alchemy is an art that once was but has now become lost to us.

Turning to the symbolic art of alchemy (inner alchemy) which has unarguably made a great contribution to human civilisation, it continues to thrive up to the present day. This form of the art seeks the refinement of the human individual through resort to often obscure mystical rituals, traditions and terminology. We have such veiled descriptions of the art as the philosophers stone, the universal solvent and the great work.

The obscure nature of alchemy in earlier times is understandable given that many of its beliefs were often in conflict with the Catholic hegemony. In those times, such conflict had serious consequences. Alchemists with their secret recipes, eathernware containers, burners, glassware and exotic ingredients appeared content to draw ridicule for their rudimentary scientific experiments if it meant escaping the ire of the Church even as they passed on their symbol-based teachings to new generations of aspirants.

In the early 1970s, educator Ivan Illich made the claim that our modern education system was the alchemy of our time. He provided much commentary on the blind belief that an education today was seen as key to special powers of wealth and influence. Curiously, one commentator who heard this noted that the man commonly known as the father of modern education, philosopher John Amos Comenius (1592-1670) of Bavaria, had also been an alchemist and there is a strong argument that his model of education was based on the principles of alchemy, namely taking the dross elements of society and refining them.

Carl Jung was one twentieth century psychiatrist who popularised the idea of alchemy as a way to self-completeness and often psychological healing and the integration of self. His teachings were based on a wide survey over decades of alchemical lore across many cultures.

I am investigating this tradition because the Chinese art of alchemy has been subsumed into the body of taiji learning and centuries of taiji practice has taken it to a new place. It has shaken out the superstitious elements and preserved and enriched the elements of value.

Simon, my teacher, would say that taiji is the fastest way for us to find our path to health and wellbeing even though, to the outsider, it looks so blunt, so lacking and seemingly so far away from what we want. Over time, I see exactly what he meant as I observe people using so much force with other methods to combine irreconcilable forces. Whereas if they let go and trusted the energy of the universe to do the heavy lifting, they would be more successful, have less side effect, be less exhausted, and be more inspired creators. It is natural for our left and right brains to work together, we don't need to train them. All we need to do is let go and stop blocking them and the rest follows from that.

The highest alchemy as I presently understand it is the blending of the form and the formless. We use the taiji form to connect to the formless energy of our being. And we use the energy of being to enrich our form. We are always interplaying physical and nonphysical. For too long, many people have lost that complete picture and rejected the physicality of life as tainted and sought some nonphysical perfection while others have reacted to them and plunged into the physical world as if this is all there is. Taiji embraces both, it rejects neither. This is why taiji is known as the pearl of Chinese culture. It is what throws a soft glowing light like nothing else can.

Taiji is a gift that continues to give. I was enchanted with the promise of taiji when I first started practising, and today I continue to look forward to my daily practice for the fresh and clear perspectives it brings me. It is a living alchemy where I can blend and harmonise and see the world from the centre of all things, not just from the physical perspective. A famous four character chengyu saying attributed to Zhang San Feng is 发财两用 （fa cai liang yong） : Both the method and material have to be employed.

Writing is an alchemy where we bring together the many threads of our experience, connect with readers, we sum up all that we know and create something new. We write new things, we read new things, this is why writing and reading are such satisfying pastimes. And so I am pleased to be able to project taiji as the art of using mind and not force.

27 Metaphysics

The principle of Ockham's Razor advises us that, in seeking to understand something, we shouldn't cut any deeper than necessary. We stay on the top line and when necessary go down to the second line and so on. Some explain it as meaning that it is futile to do with more things what can be done with fewer. I learned this principle, named after medieval theologian and philosopher William of Ockham (1287-1347), during my formal philosophy studies.

In medicine, the principle may be interpreted as meaning: 'a doctor should reject an exotic medical diagnosis when a more commonplace explanation is more likely.' It certainly makes a lot of modern day medical diagnoses and treatments seem positively medieval and in want of a lecture from William of Ockham!

For a long time, I rarely applied this principle to my taiji philosophy. I analysed and over-analysed so many aspects of taiji, especially definitions and meanings, and engaged in so much hypothetical argument, mostly inside my own head, as I swiped like a bear with bad eyesight for greater clarity about taiji. One day I realised much of my over active mind was a quest to grasp a certainty with which I could convince others. Now I know that it is not my business whether or not others accept or agree with me. Just as in my own and my teacher's original approaches to taiji, we are either attracted to it or not.

Formal philosophy has been an exhilarating activity for me. It almost cannot help itself with its constant generation of new words, new phrases, new languages and new frameworks. It is an expression of creativity at its most satisfying. As a game of intellectual swordsmanship, it is engrossing. However, except for the fun of creating, once you know the rules of the game, I question philosophy's relevance to the life of most people today. Most of us do not need to cut that deeply into the big questions to have a satisfying grasp of the nature of reality.

I do however, strongly believe that, whatever our path, it is important for us all to have a metaphysical perspective on life where I use the term 'metaphysical' in a non-formal and relaxed way, one aligned with the original sense of the word as coined by Aristotle, ie that which goes beyond physics. While we are immersed in physical reality, we need to see beyond it if we are to know how all its parts work together.

In the spirit of Ockham's Razor, this metaphysic should be as simple as possible so it is most relevant to our life and the decisions we make. There may be a better word than metaphysic, though I haven't found it yet. Consider it as a preamble to a more detailed code of living. The phrase 'spiritual beliefs' already cuts too deep as if we have left the physical world far behind. In the past, people were satisfied with the word 'religion' to encapsulate their beliefs about the nonphysical. But religions or associated philosophies often fail when they rely on distant past authority. They must be reinvented again and again to serve the people of their new day. That reinvention can never be guaranteed. We want more meaningful and relevant inspiration for who we have become, not who we once were.

When we look at a group of individual trees, we may fail to see the forest itself. That which lies beyond the physical is the matrix that holds the physical parts in their place. Some call this 'the wholeness'. Others, as we have seen, describe it as energy, an energy matrix composed of many different vibrations, a spectrum of heavy and light, going off in many directions. In fact, as long as we agree on what we are talking about we can use whatever word we like. Others will say that's where God abides.

Leibniz gave us the following description of the 'immeasurable and the eternal' to illustrate the nature of the wholeness beyond the parts:

> Look at the most lovely picture, and then cover it up, leaving uncovered only a tiny scrap of it. What else will you see there, even if you look as closely as possible, and the more so as you look nearer and nearer at hand, but a confused medley of colours, without selection, without art! And yet when you remove the covering, and look at the whole picture from the proper place, you will see that what previously seemed to you to have been aimlessly

smeared on canvas was in fact accomplished with the highest art by the author of the work.

If we accept only what we see with our own eyes, if we deny or even simply ignore the role of metaphysical forces in our lives, if we use our material world as the mirror of who we think we are, we will struggle for a clear perspective on our relationship between ourselves and our world. We will always feel smaller than we really are. And we will always be burdened by our limitations.

All of us have an intrinsic knowledge of the energy world that lies beyond our physical world. Depending on habits of thought and behaviour we develop over time, many of us overlook it, ignore it, perhaps even deny it. To choose a metaphysical perspective on the world, in the first instance, is to simply to return to that natural state where we accept that our physical and the metaphysical worlds are intertwined. To return to this state is to let go of constrictions we have imposed on ourselves as both individuals and as a society.

To hold distorted beliefs about the nature of the world will have implications: more and more, we will be shaped by those beliefs and expectations. As an example, consider a person who believes everything in life should be black and white. This is actually the application of Boolean logic which underpins a lot of our early science. It asserts that a proposition can be either true or false. The logic is that something cannot both be and not be at the same time. However, there are cases where a proposition may be partially true. It is only recently that scientists have developed a system of fuzzy logic which has led to great advances in technology. Fuzzy logic embraces the idea that in certain situations, propositions can have a truth value anywhere along the scale from 0 to 1 where 0 is false and 1 is true. The upcoming generation of quantum computers are built on the basis of such fuzzy logic.

We can all benefit from a compass to guide us through our world and we have one within us. All we need to do is to re-connect to it. This is best achieved by adopting a simplicity, often letting go, rather than doing more. It can be achieved by practices of non-doing such as meditation. There are boundless examples across human history of how people factor the metaphysical into their lives.

Human culture and civilisation is spectacularly abundant with such manifestations of religions, philosophies and other codes of thought and behaviour. Some are highly elaborate and some are austere. They all have their value. And we are free to choose any which we feel will serve us. Many have good momentum and so it makes sense to join in. Or we may wish to develop our own.

In the late nineties, when I was living in Russia, the country was in the process of recovering from seventy years of Soviet communism, a political movement based on materialism and strident atheism. The nineties saw a boom in people turning back to religion. I took the opportunity each Easter break to visit different Russian regional cities. One year I went to cities in the Golden Ring outside Moscow, widely viewed as the spiritual home of Russian Orthodox religion. Another year I visited the ancient city of Smolensk.

On each occasion, I went to the Orthodox cathedral to attend the evening service on Easter Saturday. In Orthodox cathedrals, people stand up, often for a long time. But it is an uplifting experience, with the choral singing, the chanting of ancient prayers in the candle-lit semi-darkness. Some people talk of the austere religious service in such places as a womb-like experience, fostering a rebirth of self by the end of the service.

At each service I attended, the cathedrals were full and I was moved by the range of people attending. I saw impeccably dressed wealthy men and women standing side by side with impoverished babushkas, young single people, families, people of all ages and classes of society. It was here it dawned on me how much people have a yearning for soul matters that never goes away. Attending their church serves their present deeper needs.

Perhaps communism was logically correct in its assertion that religion is outdated and irrelevant to the material concerns of the modern human being. But Marxism has always struggled to account for the human soul and its intrinsic need for a metaphysical perspective on life whatever form that may take. The tower of Marxism was built on some erroneous assumptions. While I may be inspired by the socialist dream, I differ on how we go about manifesting this dream. Again, forcing any dream will not only generate resistance, it will produce the opposite result.

If the theory has already established that capitalism carries the seeds of its own destruction, then the use of force to bring about capitalism's destruction may only be counter-productive. Of course, there may be an argument that the sooner the better to bring an end to suffering of the average worker. And that may have seemed important when Marxist theory was first formulated, but any claim that communism is devoted to the end of the suffering of the average worker is a hard one to defend today. The only real outcome of the immense application of force in Stalin's day has been to generate a desire for a better life without such force. We can manage this paradox more adeptly now than before.

On the subject of using force to promote our beliefs, I recall a funny moment during my time in Guangzhou. It was when I met some Christians who were so proud of themselves because they were smuggling bibles into China and distributing them to friends and convertees. Soon after that, I was in a bookstore in Guangzhou where I saw bibles for sale on the shelf just like any other book. Those bible smugglers may have been feeling good about their proselytising, but it was all for their sense of righteousness and little else. I wonder if they wished there was more resistance to their plans so they could feel more ennobled.

Sometimes people erect barriers in their own mind and spend too much time overcoming them without ever considering a better way. They could have spent their time and effort doing nothing, just enjoying their time, and they would have achieved the same outcome as they did with all of their needless plotting and scheming. They are hooked on forcing their message. And this can become exhausting and unhelpful. We can all find ways to use our mind more intelligently.

In summary, my attention to taiji has reminded me to look one step beyond the physical world, at the nonphysical reality, and then come back to the physical world to see how everything is in its right place. I accept that some people use a religion and some use a philosophy, and that there is always the trap that they may become too ritualistic and outdated, not serving their original purpose as well as they once did. But with a clear and open mind it is inevitable that we will find a better way.

We can always expect to see a diversity of expressions of people's metaphysical beliefs, for they will use different words and will come from different life experiences, and we know that this diversity is healthy. It acknowledges that each person has a different soul journey, and they have different needs at different points along that journey. This allows for a more dynamic social stability where respect doesn't have to be enforced because it is more easily understood and accepted.

With a clearer metaphysical underpinning to our society, we will attract governments that are less resistant to people's desires; they will rely less on restriction and enforcement and more on encouragement and independence. Under such conditions, individual health becomes a natural outcome of the environmental conditions, it becomes a by-product of a healthy society which generates less stress, causes less sense of displacement and less alienation.

Society will always produce inspired individuals who come forward with new works of science and art and new perspectives on our relationship with the world around us. Their inspirations are worth exploring as we can discover how they may enrich our own understanding of our world and how we relate to it.

28 The taiji person

Let's explore how a person trained in taiji engages with society, how he or she fits into the modern world. Be warned. There is no standard. Such a person may hang the shingle of 'master' or 'healer' outside their front door. Or they may not.

Working in a government department for nineteen years, I migrated from one work section to another every two or three years. This happened to be my personal rotation cycle. In the different areas, I worked in teams with people of many backgrounds. Being in the department responsible for driving the nation's multicultural agenda, it is understandable that we led by example. Amongst colleagues, we maintained a strong professionalism and focused on the skills required to do our job. Working close to people of diverse background and experience was the norm.

I'm a sociable type but I still marvel at often how little I knew about many work colleague's personal interests and activities outside work. I saw this as a healthy thing. We were together to get a job done and that was what mattered most. But often I would be surprised by the revelation that a close colleague had a particular artistic or technical skill or interest outside work. I discovered colleagues who were artists, musicians, singers, writers and pursued all sorts of other interests in their own time. In a similar vein, I expressed the taiji of no taiji in my professional life. That helped me do my job but was a very private thing.

It could be due to my Australian egalitarian upbringing, or it could be because of my familiarisation with French philosopher, Michel Foucault's lucid analysis of how power and language work together, each supporting the other like electromagnetic fields, that I am reluctant to use the word 'master' when referring to a highly accomplished taiji person. Or it could be the influence of my teacher, Simon, also an Australian and one who had such a sublime understanding of all aspects of taiji and held such command in any teaching situation that he would have met any definition of the term 'master' but was himself reluctant to use the word.

Simon was far more comfortable to be described as a friend, just as those people and small groups with whom he was in direct communication he would describe as friends, though perhaps in the early stages of the learning process he would refer to them as students and to himself as a teacher as a way to satisfy expectations.

In taiji, we understand that we all have the same direct access to the great dao of nature, call it the ever-expanding state of eternal satisfaction, within ourselves. And the key to finding this satisfaction is simply to manage ourselves and our own energies, and it has little to do with mastery of the world or the people around us. So our first conclusion is that we will often find taiji masters who won't carry the title of master. Their relationship with the dao is their own business alone.

A common stereotype is that great masters are often recluses, living up on a mountain, free of the cares of everyday life. I have walked several remote mountain regions in China and encountered various taiji and Daoist masters who attract followers to them, followers who are eager to learn the art in those tranquil and undisturbed places. But we shouldn't be mistaken into thinking that the typical taiji aficionado lives up on such mountains. Not a physical mountain anyway. We can see beyond the metaphor, that many have taken far too literally. Such persons, because they are so well equipped with a sense of both poise and direction, they are often successful in their life. So it is true they have climbed their own mountain of sorts. But I hope in this chapter we can dismantle that tree-covered mountain-abiding stereotype. Some may even work in shops, factories or government offices.

As did Simon, many taiji teachers engage with the world through schools and clinics. This is how they share the benefits of what they gain from taiji. I have noticed that it is a very Asian phenomenon that martial arts schools grow up around particular masters who built a name for themselves through their teaching skills. Such schools can form an important part in a student's life over a long period of time as fellow students form social bonds and treat the school as a type of second family.

As healers, many may not use the term 'healing' at all, or they will use it very cautiously because the word implies a sense of doing, of taking action to set things right, whereas the natural healer is simply about lending a hand to a person who, as part of who they already are at the core of their being, have the healing power within themselves. The best healers are often merely helping others to remove obstacles to health. They have a powerful understanding of what we call 'body wisdom'. It is not about manipulation or repair, or fighting disease. We have already established that the more we force, the more we attract resistance.

One good example is Melbourne taiji teacher, Beverly Milne, author of *Tai Chi Spirit and Essence*. I have chosen Beverly as an example of a highly accomplished taiji teacher because hers was one of the first books on taiji I read which departed from the standard taiji transmission of postures and the rights and wrongs of taiji practice. Her book includes an account of a number of innovative group exercises where students afterwards share their experience in their own words. For many years, Beverly ran both a taiji school and health clinic. She encouraged her students to use taiji as a tool to assist them in the greater path of their spiritual unfolding, each in their own way. More recently, with a stronger focus on meditation, she continues this direction of self-help and self-healing through natural means.

In the introduction to Al Huang's classic on taiji: *Embrace Tiger, Return to the Mountain*, Barry and John Stevens write:

> 'In Moah, Utah there is a tai chi short order cook who has never heard of tai chi. It's beautiful to watch him make hamburgers. In Albequerque, I knew a tai chi mailman. My father was a North of England peasant who went to London and learned a trade. He taught me to do everything without force. "Easy does it." weren't just words to him. "If you have to force it then something's wrong. Find out what it is." When I was sixteen, he taught me to drive a car, first briefly telling me the simple mechanics. After that he sat beside me while I drove, saying "Listen to the gears. Listen to the sound of tires on the road. Listen to the engine, and smell it too. Don't expect the road around the bend to be the way you think it is. Don't expect the driver of the car ahead to make any sense- maybe he's a lunatic." Be aware, alert and sensing, living and moving in harmony, with no grinding and no crash.

At its core, taiji is non-political, non-sectarian and non-resisting. So we may encounter taiji people in any walk of life. Taiji, as a philosophy, not as a martial art, is a tool for helping people to connect themselves with their greater nonphysical being. It is not prescriptive in how we should live. At the core of how these taiji people work will be a habit of doing more with the resources they have and they will achieve that with less exertion. Such people exude a firmness and gentleness both at the same time, and this carries over into their daily life.

In the early 1980s, just after I began my taiji classes, Australian actor, Jack Thompson, appeared in a television current affairs item where he was doing taiji in a snow-covered Moscow Red Square. I also recall images of an enthusiastic Jack teaching taiji moves to a host on a daytime television show. Daily taiji exercise has been one of the constants in this man's long acting career. Jack may enjoy privacy in his own home, but here is a person who has used his creative ability to support a career of uplifting a huge circle of people around the world. Through his choice of projects and his talented acting, Jack becomes part of a production team that can soothe and inspire many without him ever formally wearing the hat of teacher or healer. This is common for your average taiji enthusiast.

Given Jack's acting success, he has also lent his name to many social projects that contribute to a better society often for people who are disadvantaged. I refer here to the Jack Thompson Foundation which operates in the north of Australia seeking to skill and support indigenous workers in remote areas to build more efficient homes. This is far from the silver screen, but it is a quiet and highly effective initiative that has the potential to improve the lives of many people in remote areas through better employment and housing prospects. This is particularly important in the remote areas of northern Australia where we all need to learn how to better get along with nature, perhaps remember many valuable life skills, where expensive and ostentatious shows of force can fall very flat in the face of the harsh environment.

People are encouraged these days to monetise their skills and achievements as quickly as possible. But sometimes it's best to focus on the goal, and allow the story to unfold in its own way. It's a bit like the decision to not harvest or dig up a crop too early may lead to a bumper result later. This is again the smart application of using mind and not force in our business world.

Another interesting example of an unusual role model of a taiji person who lives on a different type of mountain, consider the former Premier of China, Mr Wen Jiabao. We have video images of him demonstrating his taiji flowing on a visit to the leaders of Japan. Wen Jiabao was known as the people's premier for the way he connected with the average Chinese citizen, and he is remembered as a politician who sought to view big policy issues for the way they impacted the lives of the average person. I have since learned that Wen Jiabao's taiji teacher, internationally acclaimed Mr Chen Zhenglei (yes, people call him a grandmaster), designed exercise routines for senior Chinese officials including President Hu Jin Tao, so they could exercise, relax and deal with the challenges of their jobs. President Hu is probably remembered as a very calm unflustered leader of the Chinese people in the first decade of the present century.

When we think about it, if we are really advocating that to use our mind more and force less is a way to a happier and more successful life, then we would expect more people in all sorts of occupations to practice taiji. However, it is a commonly held belief that people have to work hard to achieve results and it is no surprise that this ideology persists so widely.

A great case study of a high profile taiji person is businessman Jack Ma (Chinese name Ma Yun). As I write this, Ma's net worth is about $US40 billion. Most people know him through his founding of the company Ali Baba in China in 1999 that was floated on the US stock exchange in 2014.

Ma, who grew up in Hangzhou, practised English by meeting foreign tourists around the West Lake, a major tourist landmark in Hangzhou. One reason I have followed Ma's story is because of the friendship he developed with an Australian, Ken Morley, and his family after they visited Hangzhou in the early eighties. Ma visited Australia in 1985 under the invitation of the Morley family. While considering study in Australia, Ma chose to continue his study in China to become a lecturer in English and International Trade at Hangzhou Dianzi University before he set up AliBaba.

Ma was a man ahead of his time. He tells a story of how he went to a government office in Hangzhou in the mid-90s to reserve the name 'internet' for a company he wished to set up but the officials refused his request because they claimed the word did not exist in their dictionary.

Ma has long held a passion for taiji and everything to do with wu shu and martial arts. He confesses to being an avid reader of prolific Hong Kong martial arts author Louis Cha (aka Jin Yong). Louis Cha's writings are special because of the way his readership is so broad, young and old, men and women, simple and educated, so many people love his work, They savour every word he writes. He brings to incredible life old stories of valour and chivalry in China. Ma went so far in the early days of his company to encourage each employee of his company to adopt, as an office nickname, the name of their favourite character from the works of Louis Cha.

Ma began studying taiji in 1988. He has used it to maintain himself as he built his company working long and stressful hours. Ma has recently undertaken to teach taiji and to that end has set up a school Taiji Zen. He stresses that he is teaching taiji as a philosophy and not a martial art. At times he has offered a series of classes specifically for entrepreneurs.

Jack Ma's path certainly dispels any fears that to pursue an outlandish philosophy like taiji is not compatible with service to the community which rewards one richly. In late 2018, Ma announced he would step down as Chairman of Alibaba Group and become more involved in educational and philanthropic activities. Here is the path of yet another taiji enthusiast!

It is helpful to remember that the 'treasure' which the founder of taiji wished to leave with people was 'the good treasure of unified and undistracted meditation, a kind heart and utmost determination'. This will manifest in many unique ways in the lives of taiji enthusiasts.

29 Our future

'I don't think a wilderness experience is complete until it's been written about.' Ray Bane in *Going to Extremes* by Joe McGinniss

Lao Zi tells us that, while thirty spokes unite to share the hub of a wheel, it is the emptiness at the centre that makes the wheel useful. Presenting the preceding chapters, I have sought to draw the reader into the empty, though comfortable, space at the centre of this book. While my life experiences, thoughts, ideas and other moments are a series of conditions relating to my life, it is from the unconditionally empty centre, that we can see things most clearly.

In the first chapter, I mentioned that I felt I had an art that, like those Chinese paintings which had hung on my friend's wall for many years, I may have been taking for granted. Now I know that, more importantly, I have been accompanied every moment of my life by a guiding energy, call it inner being, call it god force, and it is easy to take this guidance for granted, forget how vast, how beneficial, how complete and balanced it is in how it sees us.

I share the story of my journey to encourage my fellow travellers who may, now and then, be similarly forgetful and find themselves in places of seemingly little light. When we are sucked in and carried by a culture that thrives on action at almost any cost, we can feel tired to the point of questioning what it's all about. By now, we should be aware that, if we are not ready for inspired action, non-action may well be the best option. With non-action, we gain nothing and lose nothing, but it may get us onto the best path to inspired action.

In our socially connected world, we are open to the influence of people who revel in resistance, people who who have wandered into pools of unwanted experiences and make a big fuss as they struggle to find their way back onto dry land of the wanted. I know enough about resistance and protest from personal experience. I do not deny they are valid human experiences, they are part of our formulating our better future, they are steps in the human creative process. But I also now know that we can more easily move closer to what we want this very day by a steady commitment to the use of mind more and force less.

I was instinctively attracted to taiji from an early age and have been happy to engage with it year after year. Taiji has been a wonderful instrument on my journey through this life at so many levels. It may look blunt, but it has always been sufficient. The by-products include personal health and wellbeing; it has assisted in building lifelong friendships; it has enhanced many of my professional skills; it has lent me more metaphysical understanding; and it has allowed for so much soul expression. I continue to see the benefits of tapping into the resources of our mind at the same time as I observe the futility of showy, superficial, short term solutions to so many of the personal and social problems we face today.

We hear so much about the prevalence of bullying these days. It is the horror experience for too many school children learning their way in society, too many workers just wanting to do a fair day's work for a fair day's pay, and too many people in relationships who just want to experience love. But bullying is a symptom, it is a by-product of a culture that values the use of force and believes in the need to control others. Fighting it is getting us nowhere. It has almost become an international modus operandi. We can only defuse it by coming back to ourselves and realigning our core values and fundamental understanding about our relationships with our own inner being and the world and other people. For now, perhaps the best we can do is set a good example. We need to get the metaphysics right before we can get the physical world right.

While taiji is framed as a self-defence exercise, the irony is that after we learn the art, and explore the metaphysical nature of the universe, we find we never really need to use it as a tool of self-defence. We are living in a universe that responds to our own vibration, and so by mastering our own vibration, by taking charge as the creator of our own reality, we have no need to fear others or to fight them. They are creating into their own reality, not into ours. Their world is not really any of our business. We have no need to fight with shadows. We have already established that when we are at war with another, we are actually at war with ourselves. This is the nature of human psychology.

Take the mental state of depression as an example, one of the many conditions we believe we have to fight. Unable to defeat it, many are advised it must be managed, possibly for life. But depression is just a word for a human moment in the never-ending cycle of ups and downs. It is natural that we experience those bright days and dark nights of human experience, but they come and go, all in their own rhythms. But by fixing on them and fighting them, they become a lot stickier and harder to drop.

The human mind and body have the incredible power of regeneration, something we will tap into more and more in the future. The story of the phoenix rising from the ashes is not some exotic fantasy tale; it is human experience we all have access to. I am not denying depression, but it is something to be soothed, to be nursed through till morning, when our body would normally swing into an up-cycle, actually refreshed by that down time. But to fight it, as dramatic and convincing as it sounds, is actually to bind ourselves closer to that thing we do not want. It is truly time to apply our mind to better strategies for health and wellbeing.

When I first learned taiji at Sydney University in 1980, we began and ended our exercise with a few minutes of standing meditation. At that time, all we did was to feel our breath, be aware of our hands, our feet and the top of our head. Call it taiji for beginners. Now, before and after I do taiji, I still do a few minutes of this meditation. But I also use that opportunity to feel my connection to my inner being, my nonphysical self, that great infinite thing which others express with words such as God, Dao, Nature, the Universe. I feel that this inner being is one hundred per cent present in and around me. I will never consider it to be unreachable without my need to take some special training or teaching. It has never gone away waiting for a particular condition to be met. It is an unconditional presence. It is right here, all of it, all the time. I blend with my inner being before I move and do my exercise. I also go back into a few minutes of meditation at the end of the exercise, again aware of how I am blended with my inner being, before I move into my day. I accept that I may be challenged, that I may forget just how omniscient, how omnipresent, my inner being is. I may lose this clarity in the course of my daily activities. But there is always the end of the day where I can get a good night's sleep, refresh my physical body, before the start of my new tomorrow with another round of taiji exercise. There is always gradual progress.

Meditation is such a valuable tool. Less than ten per cent of the population regularly meditates in a way that we understand meditation. However, the regular practice of meditation is one of the best pieces of advice we can offer a person. And if a person is already meditating, I would advise to make it lighter, simpler, easier. I sometimes wish I had the time to explain this to those people who come collecting money for charities. Regular meditation can do no harm and it can soothe a hundred different aches and pains of living. Meditation takes us back to a simple and direct connection with the source of our own being. Each time, that reconnection makes us feel lighter, more energetic, more focused and as if we are being reborn into the new moment. Whatever our goals, we will find new impetus to those goals even as we understand how the path so far has been one of clarification and enrichment. We understand the nature of resistance, that whether we say yes or no to something, we create more in our experience because that is what we focus our minds on, that is what we replicate.

No matter how complicated life becomes, meditation is like resolving a mathematical equation which factors in the infinite number of vector forces that are operating upon us, and they are all resolved to one simple small arrow showing us our next step. It is that simple. After any step taken, that equation with its infinite variables re-calculates the step after that and so on. It is the safest and most reliable way to move forward in the true sense of the word.

More broadly, I have observed how smart and well educated people in the modern world stumble and flounder as they grapple with a whole series of broader personal and social questions, lets call them philosophical questions, whether they be ethics, politics, psychological and so on. Even if a person has a well developed philosophical compass, it can have a flawed metaphysical basis. This is why I see a powerful need for us to develop a more relevant metaphysic for living. We know how crusty and archaic many religious traditions are in their expression of the nature of god and the world. We also see how unreliable new religions, perhaps better called cults, and alternatives can drift off course. There is no need for a taiji metaphysic, but once a person has a clearer sense of the basis relationship between the physical and nonphysical world, then a lot of other aspects of our life will often fall into place.

Zhuang Zi, in one of his stories, points out the futility of using the finite to pursue the infinite. I often think of this story when I hear people who mention the phrase: the politics of identity. If we align ourselves with a finite identity, then we will always feel incomplete, and uncomfortable. And nothing can protect us or save us. When I attended Simon's school at Canterbury, I mixed with a whole range of people of different backgrounds, gay, feminist, ethnic, alternative, disabled. Many people from particular social groups and identities have a very strong asking, for they have seen stronger contrast in their lives than others. In our taiji training, we began with the assumption that we come from the life force and we return to the life force. Boom boom. We are all equal, as energy beings. Though we can't make others understand this, we can apply it for ourselves now.

I affirm the taiji approach where, as a first step, we must let go, and immerse ourselves into the wholeness of who we really are. From there we can come back to our time and space realities and feel more able to negotiate our world. Of course, we are free to choose our company and friends and our personal pursuits. This is our irrepressible soul urge. This is the source of meaning in our lives.

I also see how the world weather and landscape is changing, particularly in a country like Australia. Much of the resistance to climate change theory is based on the claim that it amounts to a quasi-religion. There is something bigger behind the story. We have for a long time, except for a few bold individuals, seen ourselves as creatures living in this world who are subject to outside forces. This world view is supported by most religious orthodoxies. But now we are coming to a new realisation that we have an influence on our environment, and we are gaining confidence as creators of our own reality. The religious orthodoxy sees God or God equivalents as beings out there somewhere who will guide us. The new generation are riding on the back of a total paradigm shift and it is fully understandable why there would be resistance to such a big change from the older generations. As a novice conscious creator of my own reality, I now come to understand more and more that scientists, priests, politicians and teachers are merely aspects of ourselves that we have attracted. So I am more curious these days to examine and understand what I have attracted to me rather than criticise or condemn.

Returning to our enduring theme of use mind and not force, I wish to express this in terms of the concept of leverage. A lever is a mechanical device used to multiply force. Leverage is a simple way of describing the action of good taiji. Wang Zongyue once commented that other martial arts depend on the victory of the strong over the weak and the fast over the slow, they are not the result of the study of any profound art. Taiji is a profound art which employs solid scientific principles in the truest sense of the word science.

Many financial writers have written in detail about the power of leverage in the financial world. Human beings have forever sought better leverage in life. Fire and the spear were two great moments in the early human history of gaining leverage within the natural environment. Leverage is about the ability to do more with less. While history is overflowing with examples of technology which have given humanity greater leverage, the greatest lever in the world remains the human mind. This is why we need to keep it in good condition and use it the best that we can, especially when this mind is connected to the great universal mind who knows no limitation!

When we do that standing meditation at the beginning and end of our taiji exercise, we feel our feet touching the ground to experience a sense of stability. With stability, we feel the lightness at the top of our head, as if we are being suspended by a piece of string. We feel the freedom. Stability allows us to know freedom, while freedom allows us to achieve better stability. These two forces are working for each other, not against each other. We can only know this by standing in the centre and seeing how they are part of the same one great human design. This is our work. That's all.

As we face the future challenge of new technologies, it will be our collective understanding of how our lightness/freedom blends with stability/security as a whole. If we don't realise this at the basic human level, we will tangle ourselves up with more and more laws, attempting to rule with more and more force, while people, driven by a counteracting grasp for freedom, will still remind us there are no guarantees to the use of such external force and control. When we force and bulldoze and bully our way forward, we are bound to feel unsure and afraid it may all fall away at any moment.

It does sound koan-like that my inner being has always been with me, that it has always been guiding me, all the while that I was on some intellectual, some philosophical, odyssey over the decades to discover something I thought I lacked. This is the paradox of life that we all seek to manage. Some give it the name of Wittgenstein's Ladder: We are all climbing the ladder but when we get to the top, we discover that we didn't need the ladder to get there. The ladder of no ladder is the perennial paradox. This is a restatement of Lao Zi's famous Way of no Way, something we have barely begun to consciously explore as a race.

We must remember that the cycle of contrasting experiences of not knowing and then knowing is forever rich and refreshing. We are not carrying the dusty, dry past with us, rather we are creating a new moment, giving new expression to our eternal being radiating from these new times and new places. I write this after having looked back and reviewed my practice of this art over four decades. But now I am wanting to look forward, just as I did when I first began the study of this art. For in that very first taiji posture of Hand Play with the Clouds, the meditation upon the water cycle, my teacher urged us to use the exercise to ponder on the core taiji idea that life has no beginning and no end. How could we ever forget that?

Appendix One: Manifesto of Phenomenology

1 Overview

Most manifestos begin with a battle cry, a bold statement or a blooded vow, something loud and challenging, an announcement that the times are about to change forever because some great new idea has arrived and it's time for a different way of doing, that the program of all programs is about to hit the streets, and nothing will ever be the same again.

But not so here. Life will go on as usual, the world continuing to expand as it inevitably does, with some people going along with that expansion and others resisting it.

Perhaps this is more of an anti-manifesto for it's not a call for any radical new way of thinking or doing. Rather, it is a proclamation of a new way of seeing. And this new way of seeing is about going back to things themselves, without the distorted lenses of often centuries of perpetuated ignorance and/or miseducation. It is a decluttering of our mind by simply letting go of rusted and outdated ways of seeing so we can focus better in the present moment.

My goal in this project is to present to the reader the best possible book about my taiji experience as a pointer to the greater story of taiji. While I invite the reader on a journey that takes us to the heart of the subject, this is not a taiji textbook, nor is it a detailed map of taiji territory. It remains a subjective account of how taiji has revealed itself to me within my personal experience under specific circumstances. From there, I hope the reader can extrapolate beyond my circle for a better appreciation of the essential beauty and value of taiji.

To achieve this goal, I have had to seek out a suitable research framework to communicate my experience. A prescriptive or formal approach would not be suitable as I would feel too constricted in obeying rules for their own sake and that would detract from my goal: the contents would be contaminated by the container. This is not a laboratory report of a life experiment. For one thing, we cannot expect repeatability. But, also, neither is it a search for causes, explanations or justifications, nor is it a quest to win favour in the court of scientific (or philosophical) rigour.

2 Introducing phenomenology
I have therefore chosen the research method of phenomenology. This takes into account my desire for a framework of investigation which allows me to best both perceive and also describe my raw life experience, as well as to interpret it for the eventual crystallisation of knowledge and/or understanding for both myself and my reader.

The intent of phenomenology in its earliest days (the early 1900s) was a more direct and unfettered knowledge of ourselves and our world. Of course, there are many issues to be dealt with on the way towards this goal, eg the fallibility of the senses, the vagaries of memory, the impact of psychology and the influence of language. However, I am confident the method I have chosen is the best one for me to deal with the totally immersive and multidimensional subject of taiji.

The term 'phenomenology' is made up of two Greek terms: *phainomenon* and *logos*. *Phainomenon* derives from the verb 'to show oneself'. *Phainomenon* means 'that which shows itself in itself, the manifest'. *Logos* normally means 'word', 'concept' or 'thought'. Martin Heidegger translates it as 'discourse'. He also goes back to its etymology which means 'to bind together', 'to gather up' into a unity or synthesis, and 'to let something be seen'. Combining the terms as we would translate them today, we come to meaning of 'things revealing themselves for their truth or their story'.

The phenomenological method is nowadays a widely employed tool for reflective research into one's own experiences. While this tool has some key features that will be detailed below, it is a tool that will operate differently in different hands. Yet all applications of this method will be valid.

While further below I provide an overview of the theoretical aspects of phenomenology, as part of this introduction, I wish to quote here Dermot Moran (*Introduction to Phenomenology*) for the following lucid snapshot of the subject:

> Though there are a number of themes which characterise
> phenomenology, in general it never developed a set of

dogmas or sedimented into a system. It claims, first and foremost, to be a radical way of doing philosophy, a practice rather than a system. Phenomenology is best understood as a radical, anti-traditional style of philosophising, which emphasises the attempt to get to the truth of matters, to describe phenomena, in the broadest sense as whatever appears in the manner in which it appears, that is as it manifests itself to consciousness, to the experiencer. As such, phenomenology's first step is to seek to avoid all misconstructions and impositions placed on experience in advance, whether these are drawn from religious or cultural traditions, from everyday common sense, or, indeed, from science itself. Explanations are not to be imposed before the phenomena have been understood from within.

3 Historical Background

Since at least the time of Plato, each generation of human beings has grappled with notions of knowledge and truth. In all this time, when it comes to knowledge about the world, efforts have been made to resolve the seeming dilemma that we, as observers, seem in one place while the world seems to be in another place, and that world over there seems to exist independently of the observer here. We are dealing with habits of seeing, habits of thinking and the entrenchment of these habits into language. But we are reminded regularly through experience, that there is an enduring relationship between the observer and the observed. I marvel at how we, as humans, have created such a diversity of solutions to this fundamental question of the play of relationship and separateness.

In the early twentieth century, German philosopher, Edmund Husserl (1859–1938), offered a radical new way of viewing the world that challenged many classical philosophical questions up to that time. It is significant that his theories were born in the aftermath of World War One, an event that so dramatically shook the foundations of European and indeed world civilisation. Husserl's stated goal was 'to develop a new philosophical method which would lend absolute certainty to a disintegrating civilisation.'

His ground-breaking proposition which would go on to become a key plank in the philosophy of phenomenology was the notion of the intentionality of consciousness. In brief, Husserl asserted that consciousness is always consciousness of something. It makes no sense to speak of consciousness in and of itself. Subject and object are granted an essential relationship at step one of his philosophical investigation. This inherent unity will reverberate in many ways and at many levels in the body of work we today know as phenomenology.

When we look at an object, at one end of the spectrum, in the realm of pure thought, we are, in some often inexpressible way, conscious of that thing in its pure essence. At the other end of the spectrum, we are confronted with the object as it is appears, the phenomenon, and while this appearance may reflect its essence, the essence of this object of our attention may be difficult to comprehend by the use of normal scientific methods.

Phenomenologists say we need to begin with our own experience on the path to knowing the object. Phenomenology is largely about this mission of validating our experience as an essential step on that path to knowledge. We could say it is a non-logical process in that we are not imposing an external logic upon the object, but rather we are seeking to draw the logic from the object, ie part of our investigation is to adopt the pose of true observer and/or listener.

Husserl employed the ancient Greek term 'epoche' to describe this necessary initial step of any phenomenological investigation. It is a move to suspend judgement or assumptions about any object being observed. As explained above, to not do so would distort our perception. In modern words, we could say we strip the item of its labels. But as a philosophical move we say we are suspending judgment regarding the general or naive philosophical belief in the existence of the external world, and thus examine the phenomenon as it is originally given to consciousness. We adopt a presupposition-less approach. Sometimes this is described as transcendental phenomenology.

Martin Heidegger (1889-1976) developed Husserl's method and applied it to the field of metaphysics and to the question of Being. As a core concept, Heidegger asserted the concept of lifeworld (*lebenswelt*) as a state of being in the world within which we are already living and which furnishes the ground for all cognition and perception. We need to know that we and our world are a sum total that cannot be artificially divided. He criticised traditional metaphysics as seeing beings as 'things'. He also pointed out that human existence is not an entity that is simply there in the world and accessible from different points of view. But rather, human existence is some specific person's existence, it has the character of specificity. In summary, Heidegger's mission was to fathom the relationship between Being and beings. As a phenomenologist, he was not offering new propositions about the nature of things, but rather devising a new way of seeing.

Many others have carried on the phenomenological tradition and found new aspects of human activity upon which to shine its light of understanding. For example, Hans-Georg Gadamer (1900-2002), renowned teacher of hermeneutics and whose work was focused on interpretation in its many senses, defined his essential task as one of giving a proper phenomenological description of the essential human activity of understanding as ensouled in language. Gadamer characterises himself both as a phenomenologist and as an ontologist. He proposed that language does not just reflect human being but actually makes humans be, brings about human existence as a communal understanding and self-understanding experience.

Phenomenological theory has continued to develop to the present day, with new theorists focusing on the task of how to actually conduct phenomenological research. But before we look at such research methodologies, it is helpful to recap the essential purpose of phenomenology so succinctly described by French philosopher, Maurice Merleau-Ponty:

> ..to return to that world which precedes knowledge, of which knowledge always speaks, and in relation to which all every scientific schematization is an abstract and derivative sign- language, as is geography in relation to the countryside in which we have learned beforehand what a forest, a prairie or a river is.

4 Research Methodology

In the course of this work, I have discovered that the phenomenological method is closely aligned with our normal life processes of getting to know and understand ourselves and our environment. That is, it does not contradict with the process of reflection and understanding our experience that many people go through without ever having been introduced to the formalities of phenomenology.

Here I recall a book I prepared in 2007, *Tales of The Dragon, The Bear and Other Wondrous Creatures*. This was a compilation of travel newsletters I had written while working overseas from 1998 to 2007. The major focus was travel in Russia and China where I spent most of my time. My goal was to write newsletters that would be interesting to my family and friends back home. But the process of writing a newsletter was also a process of discovery for myself. And I realise now that I was employing the phenomenological method in writing each of these newsletters. Each newsletter had a different focus; the contents were a combination of descriptions of people and places, historical summaries, personal observations and experiences, collaborative efforts, and often quirky moments that could say a lot more about a place than a few pages of a travel book. I recall that one newsletter which covered my visit to both Turkey and Crimea, the newsletter was written in the first person from the point of view of the Black Sea. From this experience I understand what phenomenologists mean when they say they have no fixed method but they are guided by some important principles.

5 The practice of phenomenology: some personal guidelines

i. Phenomenology is a philosophical research method for seeing the world in an unfettered way for fresh insights, fresh meanings and new understandings;

ii. I have prepared these guidelines on how to best conduct my particular research project, but with the knowledge that there are no set rules or methods to follow.

iii. In the course of such research one usually moves through the following stages:
a. Initial engagement: Clarke Moustakas points out that any research process begins with the identification of a question that is deeply felt, a question that has an emotional effect on the researcher and cannot be ignored;
b. Immersion: A key component of our research is our raw experience. We begin with a territory of unreflective experience exactly as it stands. As part of my total experience, I have access to extensive personal resources including my own notes, scrapbooks,

books, memories and recollections and other taiji practices and memorabilia. Within the immersive stage, I observe the totality of my experience without seeking to edit or evaluate any element of it;

c.   Incubation: As per Paul Feyerabend's theory of science, the initial child-like playful activity is an important step on the path to any knowledge and understanding. While adopting the posture of immersion in my chosen experience, as I begin to consider and describe the phenomena before me, I trust that there is a sorting process happening whereby I can 'hear' the best way to deal with each element of my experience and this includes a willingness to reach out to other experiences which may not seem related to the primary research but which can better inform it;

d.   Illumination: In the course of examining and describing my experiences, I entertain new possibilities in how to relate these component experiences, and new frames of references emerge which may lead me to changes of perception towards the project as a whole;

e.   Explication: I continue to clearly examine and describe in detail my various experiences and from this significant meanings, relationships and structures emerge;

f.   Creative Synthesis: The many strands of experience and understanding that have emerged in the research are brought together to form a coherent whole.

iv. It is helpful to restate and define some key strategies in our research. Many of the following points are taken from the writings of Husserl;

v. Intentionality of Consciousness is the doctrine that every mental act is related to some object. Consciousness in itself cannot be, consciousness is always consciousness of something. This gives rise to the concept of the lifeworld, (lebensvelt) that we are forever immersed in our living environment and so cannot cut ourselves off from that.

vi. The Phenomenological Reduction is the formal term for the technique where we view phenomena in the world in a primary state of astonishment, as if we are observing these phenomena with no prior knowledge, no assumptions and no preconceptions. Husserl described it as a meditation technique where we can voluntarily sustain the awakening force of astonishment, and thus bring the 'knowing' of astonishment into our everyday experience;

vii.   To practice the epoche is to suspend our normal unquestioning faith in the reality of what we currently experience. We neutralise all judgements that posit the world in any way as actual. Effectively, we seek a change of attitude to move away from naturalistic assumptions about the world, assumptions that are both deeply embedded in our everyday behaviour towards objects and also at work in our most sophisticated natural science. An alternative description of this act is 'bracketing';

viii.   Horizontalisation: After gathering descriptions of experience, they are compiled into a list of statements and at this stage of the research, every statement is considered of equal value;

ix. Imaginative Variation: During the incubation step, in keeping an open mind for the emergence of fresh and important meanings from our research, we employ the strategy of imaginative variation in viewing our information. Here I borrow from Clarke Moustakas who has contributed greatly to models of phenomenological research, and who suggests the following possibilities in employing imaginative variation to sharpen outcomes:

a.   Vary possible meanings;

b.   Vary perspectives of the phenomenon: from different vantage points, such as opposite meanings and various roles;

c.   Free fantasy variations: consider freely the possible structural qualities or dynamics that evoke the textural qualities;

d.   Construct a list of structural qualities of the experience;

e.   Develop structural themes: cluster the structural qualities into themes;

f.   Employ universal structures as themes: time, space, relationship to self, to others; bodily concerns, causal or intentional structures;

x. Final Step: The final step in the phenomenological research process is the synthesis of meanings and essences. The essence is the condition or quality without which a thing would not be what it is: it is 'the final truth' for our relative purposes, perhaps even the title we use.

Appendix Two: Yang Chengfu's Ten Important Points

杨澄浦太极拳说十要

Ян Чэнфу 10 Требований Тайцзицюань

1 虚灵顶劲
xū líng dǐng jìn
feel empty, energised andsuspended from the halo point
усилие макушки пустотно-одухотворенное

2 含胸拔背
hán xiong bá bèi
sink the chest, expand the back
спрятать грудь, выставить спину

3 松腰
sōng yāo
relax the waist
освободить поясницу

4 分虚实
fēn xūshí
separate empty & full
разделение пустого и полного

5 沉肩坠肘
chén jiān zhuì zhǒu
sink the shoulders and drop the elbows
погружение плеч и опускание локтей

6 用意不用力
yòngyì bùyòng lì
use mind and not force
использовать намерение и не применять силу

7 上下相随
shàngxià xiāng suí
co-ordinate the upper and lower body
верх и низ следуют друг за другом

8 内外相合
nèiwài xiànghé
co-ordinate internal and external
внутреннее и внешнее друг с другом соединяются

9 相连不断
xiānglián bùduàn
continuity without breakage
связанность без разрывов

10 动中求静
dòng zhōng qiú jìng
seek stillness inside movement
b движении стремись к покою

Appendix Three: What is Opposite Meditation?

'By the delusion of the pairs of opposites,
sprung from attraction and repulsion, O Bhārata,
all beings walk this universe wholly deluded, O Parantapa.
The Bhagavad Gita VII (27)

Meditation
Most people today accept that meditation has a place in the modern world. Few would argue against the claim that the regular practice of meditation brings calmness and peace of mind.

Many people nowadays also accept that meditation can play a key role in healing our mind and body of disease. In fact, it seems that today we are rapidly heading to the realisation that the old saying *"it's all in the mind"* applies not only to how we feel but also to the world we live in.

However, integrating the practice of meditation with the activities of day-to-day living is another step again and some people can find it difficult to achieve. Those first approaching meditation may sometimes feel frustrated as they seek many of its promised benefits without a proper understanding of wholeness; even meditation has its opposite.

With an appreciation of opposite philosophy and the practice of opposite meditation, we can see how meditation and daily living can be part of the same process.

Everything has its right place
Opposite meditation is a technique for restoring our mind to its original state of wholeness. With such wholeness, we feel very content and satisfied with ourselves as we are, and yet we are also able to see clearly our best way forward to future expansion and growth.

Life has always been wholeness which, by its very nature, accepts all things and rejects nothing. In the scheme of life, everything has its right place. But our society often tries to teach us something different.

We are brought up making rule after rule about what's good and what's bad, working out what to embrace and what to reject in our belief systems, with the result that our mind can, at times, become very one-sided; we try to separate wealth from poverty, health from sickness, life from death and so on as if there was no relationship between any of these pairs of opposites.

In each case we seek to distance ourselves from those undesirable opposite poles of experience because we find it so hard to integrate them into our total life experience. Yet curiously, if we pause to look at ourselves more carefully, these opposite poles continue to dominate much of our thinking and behaviour.

Opposite meditation can work as a type of mirror. We look at ourselves from an opposite perspective to gain a clearer and more complete picture of who we are.

Opposite meditation is easy
The essence of practising opposite meditation is to take any thing or situation in mind and then imagine its opposite. For example, if it's winter and we are feeling cold, we may try to meditate on the opposite to winter, whatever we understand that to be. As we ponder on how winter becomes summer and summer becomes winter, we can see winter necessarily has its opposite which is all part of the greater natural balance. To know this can help us in the way we experience winter because we know that summer is never too far away. We can already feel the warmth of the summer which lies within us now.

Opposite meditation for health
Meditation on opposites can help ease us through many difficult situations. For example, if we are sick, we can sometimes think that we are in there so deep that there is nothing left for us but sickness. This is just the type of experience to which we can apply opposite meditation. We do this by meditating on the opposite to sickness. Then our health can become a direction for us to follow. This can even help us to better understand sickness. Backed up by good treatment and the right attitude, sickness will soon give birth to new health.

Do it your way

The way we practice opposite meditation will be unique to each of us, depending on our own experience. We may choose to visualise an opposite situation, chant a mantra such as "my opposite self", or recite a positive affirmation built around the idea of opposite philosophy, which means something important to us. They are all valid ways of practising the same thing.

Overcome blockages

There are numerous ways in which we can apply opposite meditation to improve ourselves. For another example, we may suffer from writers' block where our writing skills seem to dry up and we can't get another word out. To write down one more thing becomes an insurmountable struggle for us.

However, rather than pushing on with more and more force, it can often be even more rewarding to just let go and reflect on the opposite experience. If we could spend a few moments reflecting on what it would be like to be totally illiterate, unable to read or write, by asking ourselves what it is we would experience in this state, we may be able to find refreshing new inspiration which can liberate us from the limited circle of our own writing experience.

Handle the power

This power of the meditation of opposites has been known for ages. For example, in early China, the Emperor, on the advice of court philosophers, regularly practiced opposite meditation by imagining that he was an orphan or a refugee without any authority in the world whatsoever.

The philosopher, Lao Tzu, wrote about this. Through this practice, the emperor sought to refresh his sense of power and duty as the one with the mandate from heaven to rule the country. This was one creative way of dealing with the perennial problem of how to handle absolute power.

Gain strength through softness

Still in the Chinese tradition, the gentle health exercise of tai chi, which is practiced for health of both mind and body, is largely a meditation on the interplay of opposites.

The purpose of taiji is to develop strength through softness. Tai chi exercise looks so soft and weak the way it is practised that in some circles it is known as shadow boxing. But remarkably it is also recognised in these same circles as the self defence exercise *par excellence*. In essence, taiji exercise is a way of harnessing the benefits of opposite meditation.

Beyond us and them
The practice of opposite meditation, in one form or another, is essential if we are to enjoy total health. A danger of becoming too inflexibly one-sided in this society is that we risk becoming prisoner to the attitudes we most despise. A classic example of the effects of extreme one-sided thinking is the recent case of the anti-abortionist in the United States who murdered a doctor. The supreme irony was that, in professing to defend life at any cost, this person so willingly and knowingly took the life of another person. Meditation of opposites can help prevent such extreme behaviour by allowing us to become more complete, more rounded, in our thinking. Then we will be more tolerant of other people's points of view because we realise that their views may one day be our own.

All around the world
We have numerous examples of the value of the meditation of opposites in Western history. The Greek philosopher, Plato, went so far as to say that the opposite poles of experience were identical with each other.

Ancient Greek society regularly celebrated a Saturnalia festival where people dressed up in costumes signifying their opposite station in life. For example, rich people dressed like peasants, or the village idiot wore the clothes of the mayor. This ritual served a valuable social function of reminding people of the transitional nature of their changing roles in life. We can see it was a long-established social application of the principles of opposite meditation.

The stars have their opposites
There has long been a theory in astrology that the zodiac house in which the sun is when we are born is actually the house where the sun casts its shadow. This theory says that the most useful sun sign to guide us in un- derstanding our character is actually the sign opposite the one we normally believe to be "ours". "Our" sign is what we will one day

become if we follow the lessons laid out for us in that opposite sign. Try it!

Business
Turning again to modern times, many large companies and even government departments pay enormous amounts of money to have their staff trained to know what it's like to be a customer standing on the other side of the counter. They invest this money to either boost business or to prevent unnec- essary and costly conflict with customers. They have to do this because, as a society, we aren't consciously practicing enough opposite meditation.

A current trend in the field of business management is for managers to identify the different learning and working styles for both themselves and their staff. For example, under the Kolb theory of learning, we have four learning styles which are classified as: concrete experience, reflective observation, abstract conceptualisation and active imagination. These styles form quadrants of a never ending circle of learning. They are descriptions of how we approach new tasks and how we perform our work in general.

A common business strategy practiced these days by managers is to surround themselves with staff who have an opposite learning style. This may on the sur- face seem to make life more difficult for them. However the effect is to keep the manager more balanced, freeing them from their own subjective position to make them more whole and complete as a human manager.

Stick to the opposite
The purpose of opposite meditation is to help us to apply our meditation experience to all corners of our life so that we can gain the full benefit of our meditation experience which is meant to calm and refresh our mind and our whole being.

We can apply opposite meditation how ever we want, in any situation. The benefit each time will be an expansion of our understanding of our total life experience, and a better appreciation of our role in life and of those around us. We do this with the solid backing of the tenets of opposite philosophy which are drawn from traditions new and old, Eastern and Western.

First published in *Wellbeing* No 68 1996

Related writing

The following two works by the same author are taiji-related and serve as complementary material to the author's fuller taiji story.

Pick Up The Pearl (poetry 2016)
A collection of martial arts-focused poetry. Applying a wide range of various poetic forms including sestinas, sonnets, haiku and free verse, it is a compilation of observations, experiences, moments and exponents, covering taiji, karate, boxing, street fighting, kung fu, aikido, judo, and bagua quan as well as their underlying natural philosophies. One smashwords reviewer said about this compilation:

> '... a strong collection of non-rhyming contemporary poetry. McGowan's poems are well crafted with a sense of colloquial meter and patient mechanics, if not a simple academic approach to writing. While his works are not seemingly commercial fair, like that of most published academics, they are interesting narratives that will engage readers and hold their interest. His poetic subject matter is martial arts philosophy, which upon first hearing led me to think "Pashaw!"; but, after reading his poems and being drawn into his stories, I was pleased and enjoyed the brief time it took me to read his work. For anybody stumbling upon this book, take the time to read it. It's fun and the writing is actually good.'

TAO: Total Person and One World (articles 2007)
This is a book about the joy of healthy living through simple, natural means. It is a compilation of 19 newsletters about taiji and related subjects written over twelve years. The book contains a lot of practical information for self help health care, covering tai chi health exercise and meditation, natural healing and taoist natural philosophy. This book complements *Tales of the Bear, the Dragon and Other Wondrous Creatures*, a collection of travel stories to various parts of the world written over the same time period. There is significant reference to the essential teachings of Simon Lim, teacher and healer, who taught taiji and conducted a natural healing clinic in the Sydney region from the mid-1970s.

Other writing by Patrick McGowan

Ride A White Mare (novel 2016)
Marco Gentolini first discovers jade at a Tibetan Buddhist Temple in Bendigo. This Temple houses the largest carving of a single piece of gem quality jade in the world. The jade was imported and Marco is curious why Australian jade wasn't used. As a student journalist, he decides the story behind jade in Australia may be worth telling. Australia is said to have only low quality jade: black and dark green, with no translucent green or white which Asians value most highly. So the experts say.

On his way to a jade mine in Cowell, South Australia, Marco takes on Tom Owen, a passenger down on his luck, mostly self-made, though a person with quirky stories. Tom is more cautious in his approach to life compared to Marco, a typical Gen Y-er. As Marco and Tom seek out key people and key places in the jade game in Australia, they hear whisperings that naturally occurring white jade may indeed exist in Australia. Their quest soon becomes more earnest and their odd chemistry allows them to follow a trail of clues towards a supposedly impossible goal. They meet dead ends and false trails, but they refuse to give up.

Jade is My Stone (novel 2014)
Shipton Kingsgate is on a quest for his own special piece of jade, a stone with an illustrious history, even as the world challenges him to discover the difference between true and false in both jade and in people's hearts.

While this text reads as a novel, its thirty chapters are also a collection of stories about jade, its beauty, its history and addictive charm. The book is much like the box of jade pieces, both carved and rough, which Shipton at home likes to open and fondle from time to time, for the pleasure it brings him.

An odd collection of characters inhabit these pages. Some of them are in Shipton's own family, plus his neighbours, and his mentor, jade connoisseur, Harbie Throwley who was taught by a blind man to appraise jade. This book is a rendition of jade into words, of which even Shipton can never get enough, though of course, he can't ever rest until he finally has the real thing in his hands.

Mostly Friday Nights (verse novel 2013)
What happened on Friday nights in the Sydney suburbs in the seventies? Read these stories about Campbell and his mates from Campbelltown, told in the ottava rima style of *The Adventures of Don Juan* though with not so many heroes. Most characters in these stories are busy getting out of it. If you weren't out of it, you just weren't there. Here is a set of stories that examines the powerful asking made by your average teenager in the suburbs back in the seventies, told lovingly from the perspective of one who lived to see the expansion of life in these places as an answer to so much asking.

WARNING: These stories contain references to the use of illegal substances, underage drinking, burglary, suicide, prostitution, illicit sex, gang rape, mental illness, domestic violence, bingeing on big macs, and sex in the back of a butcher's shop. Read at your own risk.

Splitting Apart (novel 2012)
Set in the future, the 83 regions of the Russian Federation are splitting apart. A team of six in a Canberra office have been asked to provide an urgent report on the issue for their Minister. As they strive to meet their deadline, the office itself is fracturing, as personal histories surface, echoing the crisis they are being asked to report on.

Best described as a discontinuous novel, this is a story told in six parts. Each part is told in first person by a different member of the team preparing a report on the international geopolitical crisis of the break up of the Russian Federation. Nev, team leader, is ex-army, with a fixation on language for its own sake, and not real good at politics as it's played in the public service. His number two, Vic, is an ambitious, career public servant who goes after what she wants.

When Nev blocks Vic's request for a transfer, she thinks she has some dirt which will sink Nev. But Nev falls back into old habits of no-holds-barred behaviour. The story begins with Taz, the youngest in the team, and most unstable, in hospital after a work related injury. We also have Sammy, an F2M transgender, wanting to do a fair day's work for a fair day's pay, to support her family. Quinn, a former musician who joined the public service by chance works with Wes who is dealing with chronic fatigue syndrome. They all have to work together. They are all living in their own world. These worlds blend to relate a bigger story.

The Shades of Paracelsus (novel 2011)
Set in Wollongong Australia, this novel is about how the innocence and optimism of youth can be treated so shoddily, so contemptuously by the darker forces that sometimes drive big business today.

Anna Waters, 17, is a smart girl from a good home who has a passion for natural medicine. Inspired by a medieval miracle worker, she wants to bring the people of her town to healthier ways of living.

Al Flanagan, 24, a smooth talking and super ambitious businessman who works for a multinational pharmaceutical company is not going to let some reckless young schoolgirl threaten his market share or career path. But how far will he go to protect his patch?

We all wish every David could overcome their Goliath. But let's not get too romantic about this; sometimes the Davids of this world are just not patient or clever enough, or perhaps the Goliaths are just too strong. Hmmm. *The Shades of Paracelsus* is also a novel about place. It explores the Illawarra region of Australia, a place where the abrupt and unarguable logic of the escarpment meets the tireless expanse of sapphire waters of a pacific ocean. See how this place shapes the thinking of its people.

The Drain Brains (novel 2007)
The darkies: untold kilometres of storm water drains under the town. With special places like the Cathedral and the Concrete Palace, it's a world of mystery and wonder for kids who love to explore.

The Drain Brains: a secret gang of high schoolers who seek their adventure in the darkies. But they never go in there alone. And never when it rains.

Fish: the most unpopular member of the gang. Sometimes he's a real idiot. He breaks every rule you could imagine and soon ends up in deep trouble. Can Fish be saved? Or will he pay the ultimate price for being an idiot?

Can the Drain Brains remain a secret as they struggle to save Fish? And can they win against the vile and evil thing they call the Bog Monster?

www.ingramcontent.com/pod-product-compliance
Lightning Source LLC
Chambersburg PA
CBHW021617270326
41931CB00008B/742